MY MUMMY WEARS A WIG – DOES YOURS?

Michelle Williams-Huw

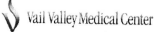

Published by Accent Press 2007

ISBN 1906125112/9781906125110

Cover design by Joëlle Brindley

Extract from *Ten-Minute Life Coach* by Fiona Harrold, © 2002 Fiona
Harrold. Reproduced by permission of Hodder and Stoughton Ltd

Extract from *The Daily Mirror* Horoscope is reproduced by kind
permission of *The Daily Mirror* / Mirrorpix

For my three boys,
my mother and father
and my sisters

*There is no such thing in anyone's life as an
unimportant day.*
Alexander Woollcott, 1887-1943

June 29, Thursday

It seems I am going to have to find out where Kylie
Minogue bought her glamorous headscarves. I have an
aggressive tumour in my right breast which will require
surgery, chemotherapy and radiotherapy, all starting in the
next few weeks. I'm either really calm or this hasn't sunk in
yet.

I had a routine mammogram for a minor complaint
called costochondritis, which is a pain that is felt in the
breast but actually stems from the rib area. I had Googled
my symptoms and diagnosed myself, but wanted it
confirmed by a medical professional. When a 'blip' turned
up on the mammogram, the hospital staff said it was
nothing to worry about. They were 99 per cent certain
everything was fine. At thirty-nine years old they don't
expect you to get cancer. Ho hum, that little one per cent
turned out to be a malignant tumour which would have
taken anything up to five years to be felt.

Everyone kept saying how lucky I was at the hospital:
Helen the breast-nurse specialist who has been assigned to
me, and Mr Monypenny, the lovely Consultant. I'm not
sure how lucky I'm feeling at the moment. The two things I
remember most about this morning are firstly, the state of
the blinds in the examination room: they needed repairing
so as I sat on the edge of the bed with my top off I was
watching people get on and off the buses outside through
the broken blind and, secondly, the five words I never really

thought I'd ever say: 'Am I going to die?'

I was on my own for the results, not thinking they would be bad. I was calm and collected when they told me, so much so that Mr Monypenny asked if I was taking it all in – then I got to the crux of it. 'You see, I just need to know, am I going to die?'

That was easy enough to say but the next bit got me. 'The thing is, I've got two small children . . . and they really need their mummy.' Tears ran down my cheeks as I spoke.

Helen the nurse gave me a tissue and the student nurse sitting by her side started crying.

'How old are they?' Mr Monypenny asked. 'Two and six', I told him. My heart was fit to explode when I uttered those words. The thought that my two beautiful little boys might lose their mummy; that their small lives might be blighted by tragedy, was too much to keep inside. They had to have their mummy – and their mummy had to have them.

Mr Monypenny told me I didn't have to decide anything now; I should go home and think about what he had said and choose whether I was going to have a mastectomy or a lumpectomy. Hello! The most major decision so far this morning was jam or Marmite on my toast; now I was being asked whether I wanted my breast cut off or not.

'You see,' I said, 'if the children are left with their father to look after them, their clothes would never be colour co-ordinated.' They laughed and it brought a momentary release.

I rang Rhodri, my husband, who was in London working, and he kept saying, 'I'm so sorry for you,' over and over. I don't know what I expected him to say, but he was sorry and I sat outside the hospital on a glorious sunny day, wanting to be a thousand miles away.

I drank a lot of wine.

June 30, Friday

As a mother myself, phoning to tell my own mother I have cancer in the same week that my father has had an operation for skin cancer (on the mouth) is a daunting prospect. It is a very strange experience having cancer, as you immediately feel responsible for the mental health of all the other people around you. My mother is one of these people. There is no right way to tell someone you have cancer; there is no way of sugaring the pill. It simply has to be said. 'Mum, I've got something to tell you. I've got breast cancer.' There it is, out there.

If I found out one of my own children had anything wrong with them as serious as this, no matter what age they were, I think it would be one of the worst imaginable situations. Mum was obviously shocked, as was my father, chipping in from the background, saying uncharacteristic things like, 'We'll support you,' (when they were about to leave for the hospital to see if he would get the all-clear for his own skin cancer). Bloody hell, we're all riddled with it.

My mother was practical and supportive in the way only a mother can be when one of her children is ill – although I don't, of course, *feel* ill. As I keep saying to everyone, 'I feel fine'. I am fine – apart from the cancer. It's the old story: go into hospital a healthy specimen, come out with a life-threatening condition, ho hum.

Twenty minutes later, my mother rang back. 'Shelley, it's Mum here. Me and your dad have had a chat and we've completely come to terms with your cancer.'

I laughed. 'What, in twenty minutes?'

'Yes,' she said, 'we're fine now, we're over that.'

Great. Let's hope it takes me as short a time to come to terms with it.

Mum rang again later, to tell me Dad had the all-clear on his skin cancer.

'How is he?' I asked.

3

'Forget about him now,' Mum said. 'It's you we're thinking of.'

'Yes,' I joked. 'I've got worse cancer than him – I've trumped his cancer.' She did laugh but I know she was hurting.

Helen the breast nurse came to the house today. Whoever doubted the NHS? I've only had wonderful service – now I know why I pay those enormous taxes. She was with a student nurse – the one who had cried the day before. At one point I think the student nurse actually fell asleep. It was rather surreal and I'm sure a less robust person than myself would have found it upsetting, but I thought it was very typical of my life in general. Nothing is ever straightforward, plus I forgave her as she had cried when I was talking about my children when I had my diagnosis. Also, I remembered what it was like to be a student myself.

Helen came to discuss my options because, 'Let's not forget who's in control of the situation here – you,' she said reassuringly. Oh yes, I really feel as if I am in control. One minute I'm leading my tra la la life, the next minute someone is asking me whether I want my breast cut off.

My options are lumpectomy and sentinel node biopsy, or mastectomy with sentinel node biopsy. My reaction is to have a mastectomy like Babs, my friend who has recently had a double mastectomy. That way, I will never have to think about the cancer again – it's gone, that's it. Or so I thought. Apparently, cancer doesn't work like that.

It's not as straightforward as taking your breast off and the disease never coming back. If the cancer does come back, it can attach itself to the wall of the chest. Oh my God, these are issues I have never wanted to think about in my life. Babs, I have since discovered, had cancer *in situ*, which means it wasn't going anywhere, whereas I have an aggressive tumour which most definitely does go somewhere, and if it's not caught in time, that somewhere is usually one's vital organs; and basically, I think by that point you are fucked.

Sentinel node biopsy is a procedure they don't do all over the country; they inject you with a blue dye that finds the main nodes under your arm. They take these away and see if they have any cancer in them. If they do, they take all of the lymph glands away. If they don't, you get to keep them.

I asked how accurate it was and Helen said about 96 per cent so I decided to go for it – option one sorted. As far as option two was concerned, I decided to have the lump removed and see if they could get clearance around it; the doctors have to have a certain circumference around it to make sure it doesn't come back. I will then have chemotherapy and radiotherapy after the operation.

Mr Monypenny is apparently one of the pioneers of sentinel node biopsy and breast surgery. Helen says the team of surgeons at the hospital are at the forefront of pioneering surgery, and I secretly wonder if all breast nurses across the country say this. She has worked for My Monypenny for years and says he's a perfectionist. Well, that suits me. As a control freak perfectionist myself, this is a big plus point in his favour.

When it's time for her to go, Helen gives me a pile of booklets and papers, and tells me to call her at any time. As she leaves, she rolls her eyes at me over the student nurse – who by this point is sitting in the front garden.

I asked Helen if I could have my op after our summer holiday in Brittany, which is the last week in July and first week in August. She said that was fine and it would be early August. I want to spend that time with Rhodri and the children before it all kicks off. We've all really been looking forward to the trip and Elis, my older child, would know something was up for sure if we didn't go.

I also asked if she thought the cancer might go out of control before I came back, because I didn't want to delay my operation for a holiday if it meant my life being cut short. Apparently, cancer doesn't work like that. I am finding out a lot about how cancer does and does not work.

Life at home carries on as normal. There are dishes to wash, children to bath, nappies to change, food to buy. We don't mention breast cancer (BC as Rhodri and I refer to it in conversation) in front of Elis. I don't want to frighten him, don't want him to think there's anything wrong with Mummy in any way. Osh is away with the fairies and doesn't know what time of day it is, so it's not an issue with him. The phone hasn't stopped ringing. I've told my story about fifteen times and my head is spinning a little.

It was Elis's sports day today; I missed it but Rhodri went. I couldn't face talking to people in a happy jolly voice knowing I have breast cancer. Elis came second in his race – he told me this morning he would either come first or second, not boastfully, but in a 'that's just the way it is' type of voice. I said second was brilliant, but he wasn't having any of it. My God, he is like me – I have gone to great pains to keep him from being the obsessive perfectionist that I am, and now look.

I drank a lot of wine.

July 2, Sunday

I have spoken to all my sisters now. I am one of four girls. My three sisters are Joanne, the eldest, then Julia, then me, then Sarah. We have always been very close and I know they will be there to help me through this. The weekend was mad, with people getting in touch. Rhodri's mother was very emotional on the phone as expected and, like my mother, said she would have the cancer for me if she could. I am not sure I would want to live with the guilt of giving this to anyone. I called Ben and Bree and Ian J, as we are having a farewell dinner on Saturday. Ben and Bree and their baby Nancy are moving to Brighton.

We have all been looking forward to going out for weeks. My mother had the children (having cancer gives you umpteen instant offers of babysitting). I didn't want to be a party-pooper on the night so got it out of the way, by phone, before we saw them. We all cried and said we loved each other. I've been doing a lot of that this weekend – mainly in a drunken haze. We had a fab meal and talked about the cancer but also didn't talk about it and the evening wasn't spoilt by it, because I wasn't going to allow it to. I keep saying to everyone how positive I am because the doctors caught it early.

We laughed and talked about the last eight years we've all known each other – God, eight years have gone by in the bat of an eyelid. We had a lovely evening, drank loads of wine and went back to Ian J's house, where Rhodri and I stayed over, as I couldn't move off his sofa.

Ben and Bree left about twelve – it was their first night out together since baby Nancy was born seven months ago. Bree called me a few weeks ago and said she just wanted the five of us to all go out, like we used to before we had commitments and babies. 'I just want it to be like it was,' she said, but the truth is that none of us will ever be those people again: we've all grown up and no one noticed. We are parents and homeowners and we've all got jobs with responsibilities – and I've got cancer and I will never be the same again.

July 3, Monday

My boss, Martyn, who I thought would find the whole business of discussing intimate parts of my body in a rational manner excruciating, has been wonderful. He has two sisters-in-law who have had breast cancer; one of them has died of it – not a good story – and one of them hasn't and is living to tell the tale – a good story – so he is well versed in diagnosis, prognosis, treatments and outcomes.

Clare, our boss, was great too. She asked me into her office and was really supportive and helpful, and I was all positive and felt somehow quite grown-up. She has said I must take whatever time off I need and not think about work. Of course, I didn't actually say that my work had become small and trivial at this moment, but I think she knew, and I was grateful for her understanding.

Emily and Paul in the office have also been very kind. It's quite unusual to see people so shocked about yourself; not in a 'You are having a baby!' kind of way but in a 'that's bloody awful!' way, and talking to you quietly as you talk to someone whose parent has died or something. Paul's girlfriend has had breast cancer twice – *twice*, bloody hell – so he was particularly knowledgeable about it.

July 5, Wednesday

I'm counting the days until our holiday. Luckily, it's not too hectic at work and I am attempting to put things in their rightful place. Some poor bugger has to come and find some order in this mess when I am away, and I will be away for about six months. It's slightly perverse, but having six months off work doesn't seem too bad a prospect.

Yes, I know I have cancer, but if having six months off is what I need to get through it, then so be it. I am spending a large amount of time Googling breast-cancer sites, gathering as much info as I can. I am fast becoming an expert. Give me another year and I can probably start practising alongside the lovely Mr Monypenny.

The phone doesn't stop ringing at night, it's constant. I am getting a bit tired of telling my story now and I want a rest. I would quite like to go back to the quiet, noncancerous me who had a few phone calls and went out and had friends round and didn't have to think about whether I was going to live or die, or keep my breasts or cut them off. Didn't have to wonder whether my husband would get a new wife within six months of me dying, or whether Osian will remember me when he grows up if I die now, or whether Elis will remember all the lovely moments we've had together or the shouty, irritable mummy moments and how sad everyone would be when I died, blighting his beautiful, young life.

July 12, Wednesday

Today is Elis's end-of-year play. Firstly, I do like Elis's school. It's a small Welsh-language school slap-bang in the middle of a city, Cardiff, but it feels as if it's in rural Wales.

For a lot of people growing up in Wales – myself included – we came here for a better life, but we still want to bring our valleys' ways or, in the case of the school, our very old-fashioned, high moral values, usually associated with rural Wales, with us, and there is NOTHING wrong with that.

The play involves every child in the school, and that's about 180 children, and is nothing short of a piece of nationalist propaganda, which I think is bloody great, because if we're not teaching them at six that the English drowned Tryweryn or that people threatened to go on hunger strike if we didn't get our own Welsh language TV channel and that, I quote, 'The story of the English is not the Welshman's story' then you are fucked, because the only way the bloody language is going to survive is if these children believe that they are special, and that people before them have been denied the right to speak the language so they need to keep that right and that language alive.

That's why I fell in love with a first-language Welsh

speaker who is passionate about his country and his language and who once spent a night in jail through protesting and that's why I want my children to speak Welsh. I feel I was robbed of my language and am glad that my children will never grow up feeling that they were denied a language that is rightfully theirs. I just wish the play was a bit shorter than two hours.

Sitting through those two hours on a child's chair, which was clearly too small for my big arse – so much so that a bit of it was on the chair of the bloke next to me – has made me realise I've no excuse now not to learn. I've got six months off coming up – the ideal time to have a go. The first time I tried, work commitments stopped me, and the second time I was pregnant and didn't have any brain cells left. I can understand lots of Welsh, however, and speak a little, and I've got Elis to practise with (Rhodri's Welsh is odd and too fast), plus I can teach Osh as I go along.

I will find out about Welsh classes, and this time I WILL LEARN and I will return to my employer, the BBC, a greater asset than I surely already am.

July 14, Friday

Osh is in the crèche today. Normally he is at home on Fridays but I'm having some 'me' time. I always feel a little bit at sea these days when I have 'me' time. My 'me' time usually involves me manically tidying the house, watching a bit of Paramount comedy, cooking something wholesome for the family – in this case a shepherd's pie – and then wondering what the bloody hell I did with my life before I had children and a husband. Well, I had lots of friends who I would meet for coffee, then we would go out to eat or to the cinema or the theatre. We would usually get drunk so the next day was a bit of a write-off, but that didn't matter too much as we didn't have any children jumping on our heads at 7.30 in the morning demanding to be fed and watered. Ah, those days . . . Actually, I don't miss them. Give me what I've got – really, I mean it. In fact, that whole single thing would scare the shit out of me so I hope to God Rhodri doesn't leave mel.

Actually I wouldn't bother again, PLUS let's look on the bright side: I might die of cancer so the singles market may never be an issue for me, unless there's something going on in heaven or down there in the other place, or limbo or wherever Buddhists go. I suppose if you believe in reincarnation you might come back as an animal, and they don't even have to observe the social niceties. They just jump on each other's back when they are in heat and shag the living daylights out of each other.

Men never have any problem with their 'me' time, do they? As most of their bloody lives are spent having 'me' time, they are never at a loss as to what to do with it.

The sound of silence around me, the stillness, the calm in this empty house, can almost be felt. When I was here alone at first, I always had something on – the radio or the telly, or I was phoning people. Now I want the silence, although I still crave the noise and the smells of cooking and the episode of *Scooby Doo* I could repeat verbatim. I want them and yet I don't.

July 15, Saturday

This evening, I went to the Spar shop to get some wine. I have always liked a drink, and drinking is linked to breast cancer. I think that is why I was not surprised when they said I had it. I am ticking lots of 'how to get cancer' boxes: I've had children late in life, I never breastfed and I drink wine several times a week, so I'm up there on the 'Things Not To Do' list. My cousin died of breast cancer at the age of forty-six and she left an eight-year-old son; my aunt by marriage also died of breast cancer and she left four children: that's five children in my extended family who have grown up without their mummies because of breast cancer.

The Spar is near Llandaff Cathedral – a beautiful place. I am not religious *per se*, but I do believe in something. You can't watch Colin Fry and NOT think there is a spiritual dimension in life, a place where people pass to. I have also seen a ghost. When I was a student I was woken up one night by a blue flashing light outside my window. An elderly man, Len, and his lodger, Andrew, who was about twenty-five, lived next door. Kate, who I shared a flat with at the time, liked Andrew and used to chat with him. She had once reported a break-in in his van to the police; they caught the people who did it and he came round with some flowers for her.

Anyway, they brought a body out on a stretcher in a body bag. I thought that it was Andrew because Len stood outside the door and, as they took the body past him he extended his arm as if to say, 'This way.' The next morning I found out that it wasn't Andrew who had died, but Len. Len was in the body bag, but I had clearly seen him in the doorway, so I know that there is something. I know what I saw and I had seen Len with my own two eyes when he was dead.

When I was waiting to go for the mammogram, Rhodri was away. I was in the hallway about to climb the stairs with a pile of washing in my hands, late one night, when I started thinking about my babies and life without them, and I got down on my knees there and then and prayed to God to save me, not for myself but for my babies.

You never find an atheist on a sinking ship. I did not make any pacts with God but selfishly asked for myself. I thought that maybe God would not like it – me being selfish and asking him to save me – that it was cowardly, but it was so spontaneous and, I suppose, so desperate that I did it.

I have never mentioned this to anyone, until now. Perhaps this is God's way of testing me, or maybe I should just be grateful that my breast cancer is at an early stage and that if I get through this, I may be a better person – maybe that's what I should aim for.

The cathedral door was shut so I sat in the graveyard and contemplated life and thought what an amazing evening it was. A group of American tourists passed by and a woman smiled at me the way someone smiles at you when they think you are in a graveyard because you have lost someone. I suppose I have lost someone; someone has died that I knew and that's me. I am no longer that person – that person is gone. I am a different person now and I must try to be a better one. I need to learn to speak my mind when I feel things are not right and to hold my breath and count to ten when I want to shout at my children, or belittle Rhodri just because I can.

Rhodri is really only a baby: he's four years younger than me, quite immature at the best of times, and I wonder if he will ever be able to give me what I want, as I go through this. I love him with all my heart, I truly do, and I couldn't wish for a better father for my children, but in truth we have little in common apart from the children and a bloody great big mortgage. Where have those two people gone, who couldn't keep their hands and eyes off each other? I want them back, I want them together again. There are occasions when I see glimpses of those people, but they are few and far between.

Kate's husband left her and now has another woman, and that knocked me for six (never mind what it did to Kate). I thought they were rock solid; that they were the together-for-ever type and then he ups and leaves after ten years of their relationship: the same amount of time Rhodri and I have been together. You think, What the hell was that about, those ten years together just gone like that? What if that happened to us?

Rhodri has plenty of opportunities to have affairs. He's never bloody well here for one thing, he travels all the time with work, and when you're in another country, how does anyone else know what you're up to? He could have been unfaithful to me for the last ten years and I would have known nothing about it. I keep asking him if he'll ever leave me and he says, 'Why would I want to leave you? You're a goddess, you're amazing.' Then I think, I expect that's what other men say to their wives and then bugger off with another woman leaving their relationships and their children.

Elis often asks me when Rhodri and I are going to have two houses because he knows quite a few friends who have divorced parents and I think he views it as a progression in life, something that happens. I explained to him that some people don't get on with each other and they shout a lot and it's sometimes better if they live in different houses. His reply was, 'You and Rhodri are always shouting at each other.' Hmm, I can't argue with that one. He also says, every time I explain why people divorce, 'But they still love each other, Mum, don't they?' Well, sometimes they don't but at his age he thinks love is a thing that you have for ever and why would he think any differently? I hope he never has his beautiful heart broken – otherwise she'll have me to answer to.

I went home and drank the wine with Rhodri and went to bed and sobbed my sad little heart out to him, repeating over and over again, 'I don't want it, I just want it to go away, please make it go away.'

July 17, Monday

Work is still manic. Andrea, who took over for six months when I was on maternity leave with Osh, will be taking over again. I can't quite make out if she was seconded under duress, or whether she actually wants to do it. We're also having Jean, who was doing little bits of work for us, to answer the phones and generally help around the office, so things should be OK.

July 19, Wednesday

I rang the hospital today to ask for my appointment date so that I could 'plan my entire life around it' as I said to Mr Monypenny's secretary. My date is 9 August, two days before I was due to go back to work after my holidays. Clare came in to see me and has agreed that I don't need to come back, so I can 'prepare' myself for the op. 'Preparing' myself in reality means running round like a blue-arsed fly making sure everything is done in the house and arranging for my mother to look after the children. It's good that it will still be the school holidays so Elis won't have to be in school.

Rhodri is due to work on the ninth and my mother has suggested – well, said – as she doesn't really do suggesting – that Rhodri sticks to his routine in work. Originally, he agreed, but now he says he thinks he should not do one of the Proms that he was due to direct. He asked me if I wanted him to be there with me and I said, yes, I did. The problem with Rhodri's job as a TV director is that it is a big deal for him to have to get someone else to do his work. There's so much preparation and it is difficult to find people at short notice, but I suppose your wife having an operation for breast cancer is also a big deal, and for once I want to be put first – before football and work, or work and football, which are interchangeable but always at the number one and two spots.

July 20, Thursday

Babs has come to see me with Dr Susan Love's *Breast Book*. Yes, she is a real doctor and yes, that is a real book. Suddenly a whole new world of research has opened up for me. Babs has recently had a double mastectomy so I feel well versed in aspects of breast cancer and surgery, having talked it through with her over the last six months. I met Babs when I did my masters degree seven years ago; we did our masters degrees together, we got pregnant at the same time, and then I rang her up four months after her mastectomy to tell her that I too have cancer.

We just seem to have these life-changing moments at around the same time. I have told her I am waiting for her to win the lottery as I know that I will be guaranteed to win too. Apparently, she doesn't do the lottery – unlike me with my standing order with Camelot. I've told her she has to start buying tickets.

Babs is the reason I went to the doctor in the first place. Even though Mr Monypenny and Helen said I wouldn't have been able to know I had a tumour, I am convinced that I did know. I knew there was something and that is why I went to my GP three times. We have learned to rely on medical technology so much that sometimes we don't listen and respond to our own thoughts and feelings about our bodies. Finally, I went to see a locum doctor and she referred me. I told her that my friend had had a double mastectomy and, even though she thought it was nothing to worry about (her husband was a breast surgeon), she said she would refer me to put my mind at rest. That woman probably saved my life just by wanting to put my mind at rest. Thank you.

I have become obsessed with Susan Love's book. There are those in life who are information gatherers and those who are information avoiders: I am the former. In fact, I would go as far as to say 'I love Susan Love.' Her practical,

16

'OK, you've got cancer, so let's look at the options here,' is really what I need at this moment in time.

July 21, Friday

Holiday, it will be so nice (sung to Madonna tune). *We're all going on a summer holiday* (sung with Cliff Richard lilt). Oh my God, I so love being on holiday and what's more I don't have to go back to work. I know I shouldn't be happy about that, but work has seemed so trivial. I just feel that I need to get out there and live a bit of life and be with my children on beaches looking in rock pools and eating ice creams.

We arrived in Roscoff, and are staying one night at a hotel in the town. Roscoff is a beautiful little port town and the weather is fab here. We went to a restaurant and all sat down, including Osh, which is unheard of – he can't sit on his arse for more than five minutes usually. We had pizzas and wine and lemonade, and to all the world were like a 'normal' family. I often wonder if other families, when they manage to sit in a restaurant without the parents having a row, the children having a row with one of the parents or the children having a row with each other, when somehow it all comes together and no one rows or runs about. Do they sit there thinking, Hurrah! We are to all the world like a normal family?

I texted my sister Sarah in Ireland and said we were sitting down having a pizza and we were like a normal family. She then texted my other sister Julia in Wales saying that I was sad, obviously thinking that I meant we looked like a normal family but in fact we were a family blighted by tragedy and had a cancerous mother who was trying to keep it all together – while sitting overlooking the harbour with two exceptionally well-behaved children and a setting sun. So Julia texted me to ask if I was OK saying that Sarah had said I was sad. I said Sarah had got the wrong end of the stick, with my text, so then Julia texted her and I texted her, by which time our pizzas had been devoured and we were on to the ice-cream part of the evening.

The hotel room had two double beds in it and we'd set up the cot for Osh. As we walked back from the restaurant I said to Elis, 'Ooh, lucky you, you'll have a bed all to yourself.'

'Oh no,' he said, 'I'll have to sleep with you or Rhodri.' He has always called his father Rhodri since he could speak, for some reason.

'Who is it going to be then,' I said. 'You choose.' Thinking of course it would be me.

'OK, Mum,' he said, 'the next time we are in France and we are in a hotel room with two beds, I'll sleep with you.'

Ooh, he really should be in the Diplomatic Service, that one. I didn't mind a bit that he was going to sleep with Rhodri as he wriggles and hogs all the bed, so I was in a hotel room in a double bed all by myself.

July 22, Saturday

The camp site is very nice, with three swimming pools, a bouncy castle – Rhodri and I will be on that later after a few drinks – a club house and a park nearby. There's a little harbour and some amazing rock formations and, better still, we are the *only* English-speaking family on the site, which is mainly Dutch and French. Rhodri and I love going to places where you don't hear anyone speak English as then we feel that we are 'real' tourists. God knows how we ended up in this place though, we found it on the internet.

We once stayed in a place in Spain and only heard one other English couple all the time we were there. Rhodri whispered, 'There's Brummies on the beach,' so we moved along the beach – not that I have anything against Brummies *per se*, we just wanted to think we were special. And if they were near us we talked in Welsh, which proved a bit difficult as I am at my most fluent when I talk about the weather; anything slightly more complicated than that is a problem.

July 23, Sunday

I am in semi-paranoid mode as there is a decking sun terrace outside the caravan and Osh cannot be trusted to stay outside on his own. He wanders off and there are cars going past occasionally. It only takes one knock and that is it: he is dead. Rhodri is in his relaxed holiday mode which does not involve thinking about the dangers that a six year old and a two year old could encounter in a strange place. He keeps saying very annoyingly, 'They're fine, Shell.' This being relaxed extends to Osh being left on the sun terrace – which I have said categorically can not happen, and to reading a book while Elis is in the pool.

I don't mind Elis going in the pool by himself – that is, after all, why we have spent the last twenty weeks driving him to swimming lessons every Monday night, so that he could actually make a decent attempt at saving himself should he fall in the water. But there are lots of children there jumping into the water which comes over Elis's head and, while he could save himself in an empty swimming pool, if one of those testosterone-fuelled teenagers jumped on his head – which is a possibility because they are all jumping in like maniacs – then he would be in trouble. I know the chances of this are remote and I know it's a pain to have to monitor Osh every minute of the day, but we are their parents and it's our job to keep them out of danger while still trying to give them a good time, and Rhodri saying, 'They're fine, Shell,' is not going to wash with me.

This means that I am constantly on Rhodri's case as I can't be in two places at the same time and he just has to accept that coming on holiday is about them, not about us sitting down to read our books. How many stories have I read in newspapers about children getting killed on holiday because the truth is, *that*'s when our guard is down. But it should be doubled because the possibility of something going wrong IS REAL, RHODRI. At least the wine is cheap and nice so I'm looking on the bright side.

July 24, Monday

Have period from hell. Am feeling a bit frazzled. Rhodri said he'd take the boys to the beach and I could meet him later so I could sit down and read a book and have five minutes to myself. I agree and then think, Oh my God, I've let him go to the beach with the two of them. Will I ever see any of them alive again? This is only day four of the holiday; please tell me that other mothers are like this. I start reading my book, *The Kite Runner*, which is really captivating so for a while I do forget that I am a paranoid ball of stress and that my children may not make it to the end of the holiday in one piece, or my marriage for that matter.

I go to meet Rhodri at the beach a bit later. It's about a ten-minute walk and when I arrive, I cannot believe my eyes. It is the most beautiful beach I've ever seen – miles of sand with very few people on it, big rocks and rock pools, some swings, and it's all so clean. There's not a single bit of litter anywhere and it's not because they have people picking it up, it's because French people are bloody civilised and take their rubbish home with them or put it in the bin.

Ahh, it's heavenly here. I started walking up the beach looking for a man with two small children and a red pushchair. Not a great feat, you would think, but half an hour later I'm still looking. I have already approached two men with two small children and red pushchairs. One I was so convinced was Rhodri (although I didn't have my glasses on at the time) that I sat down next to him. It's a wonder he didn't get the French police out as I must have seemed very strange – good job I didn't start taking the baby out of the pushchair! Anyway, I eventually found them (about five feet from where I started in the first place), looking all happy and sunny and pleased about the beach, as if they had discovered America.

July 27, Thursday

The period from hell continues. It is impossible for me to contemplate swimming, so I sit by the edge of the pool, never taking my eyes off Elis. The pools are lovely, but deep, over my head in places, and Elis has much more confidence than ability. God, how old will they have to be before I am sitting by the side of a pool sipping a cocktail and not worrying myself into an even earlier grave than cancer could put me in, wondering whether they will make it to the end of the fortnight? Am I mental? I see danger everywhere and I just feel that Rhodri is lackadaisical about their safety. If anything ever happened to either of them, my life would not be worth living.

July 28, Friday

This place is lovely. I'm trying to calm down a bit; maybe it's just the whole cancer thing that is making me so bloody edgy. I am reading *The Breast Cancer Prevention and Recovery Diet* book by Suzannah Olivier, and Dr Susan Love's *Breast Book* as I need to clue myself up on everything, but they serve only to remind me of my situation and Susan Love's book can be a bit scary, to be honest. Went out for a pizza earlier as there are only so many super food salads, as recommended by Suzannah Olivier, a couple can take in one holiday.

Bretons love children, and they don't look at you as if you have two heads when your child starts getting a bit naughty in a restaurant. Just as well really, as when Osh takes it upon himself to run about it is very difficult to keep him in his chair. Oh well, next year he'll be older and not so much trouble, and might actually sit down for more than ten minutes.

July 29, Saturday

Sue and Mario and their two children Ollie and Lewis (Sue works with Rhodri) are in Brittany at the same time as us and we all met up for the day. We drove about an hour and they drove about an hour. It was just perfect; the weather had been a bit overcast but when we got there the sun came out and we all went into a restaurant on the sea front and had a meal, and all four children behaved like normal children. They sat down and ate their food perfectly – the God of Mealtimes was looking down on us once again. We went on the beach for the day and the children ran in and out of the water like mad things.

Rhodri and I have been playing a trivia quiz most nights since we arrived. We are also only drinking one bottle of wine a night between us; this is unheard of, but it means that for once in my life I am sober when I am doing the quiz and I keep winning. I can tell that Rhodri just can't believe it and he keeps saying in a very patronising voice, 'well done, Shell,' just like I'd say to Elis if he managed to actually draw something that was recognisable. Rhodri can't stand it that I am better at something than he is. He grew up mainly watching Welsh language telly and his cultural references are different from mine – I am excusing his lack of trivia knowledge now. Also, I am very good at retaining relatively useless pieces of information that serve neither man nor beast unless they are the answer to a trivia question. No matter – I feel all superior and clever.

July 30, Sunday

Spent the day on the beach. I think I am a pervert. There is a lifeguard there who is a Brad Pitt look-alike. I think he might actually have some inkling that he is sex on legs as he is ever so slightly peacocky, in a cool way, though. God knows how old he is, it's difficult to tell – in his late twenties I guess. Behind the anonymity of my sunglasses I am shamelessly ogling him – it's hard not to – you would not be human if you didn't notice how gorgeous and how full of vitality and hormones he is. I am Mrs Robinson!

Not, of course, that he would ever even notice me in my size 14 Marks & Spencer swimsuit, which I guess is a good cover, as he wouldn't think I'd be perving him up as he was looking out to sea for people to rescue. I am sure there was a time when I would have been desirable to a man like French Brad, but that really was a long time ago. Oooh, maybe I should get into 'difficulties' so he can come and rescue me. I will try to lose about two stone and buy a new swimsuit first, though. Surely that is achievable within the next four days or so?

July 31, Monday

Kerry has had her baby by C Section. Baby Daisy. Richard C rang to tell us. Mother and baby doing well. Unzip them and get them out – I'm all for it.

August 1, Tuesday

I feel so alone. Last night I finished reading *The Kite Runner* – a book that is not for the faint-hearted and certainly not for someone like me who is verging on the edge of a nervous breakdown. Anyway, I was sobbing when I finished reading it, and it became something of a release for me as I haven't really cried about myself. Rhodri had already gone to bed and was sleeping so I slipped into bed to be with him, and I woke him up and said, 'I was reading *The Kite Runner* and it was so sad,' and then I blurted out, 'I don't want to die,' and I was crying and he mumbled, 'I'm really tired, you woke me up.'

I am confronting my worst nightmares and my husband tells me he is tired. I couldn't believe it! He is so bloody selfish – he does not have a clue what is going on in my head. He is wrapped up in himself and the only thing he cares about is how anything affects him. He is emotionally stunted, he always has been. I don't know why I expected him to miraculously change overnight just because I have cancer. I left the bedroom, I couldn't speak, I was crying so hard and went to sleep in with Elis. I hated Rhodri at that point, I just hated him, and I thought I could never forgive him for not being there in my darkest hour.

He came into the bedroom and said, 'Look, I'm sorry, I'm really sorry, you woke me up and I didn't know what I was saying,' which I think is crap. I think he knew exactly what he was saying; he just thought, Shit I shouldn't have said that. Whether it was because I wanted to believe him or because I didn't want to be alone and needed the touch of another person, I went back to bed with him but I am wounded by it and don't think I will ever be able to forget it. I feel as if I have no one I can talk to, and that's it. I don't want to die; I want to live and I wish this would all just go away.

August 2, Wednesday

Went to a children's play park today called the Parc du Loisirs which Rhodri and I kept referring to as the Parc du Losers which upset Elis and we had to be quiet as he said he didn't want to be in a park for losers. He's just like his father – no sense of humour. Osh and a little French boy kept going up and down this slide which had some steep steps. The little boy's father kept helping Osh up – God, he was gorgeous, tall, dark and handsome and French, that bloody accent just sends me crazy. His wife was so thin.

I'm always looking at wives of handsome men, hoping they are a size fourteen to sixteen but they never are. All the women smoke in France; that's why they are so thin. Although I have a handsome husband and I'm not thin. I wonder if there are French women looking at my husband and then looking to see if he has a thin wife and spotting me and thinking, What's he doing with her?, except they would be thinking it in French and I have lost my French phrasebook, so can't translate that.

I have discussed with Rhodri telling Elis about my operation. I want to tell him because he will pick up on it or will hear someone talking about it, but I don't want him to be freaked out about it and think there is something terrible wrong with his mummy. Shit, actually there is something terrible wrong with his mummy. It is just easy to put this at the back of my mind in this place as everything is so normal and nothing has actually happened yet.

Elis and I were lying on the beach, Rhodri had taken Osh off for a walk and I said, 'Mummy needs to have an operation on her booby. There is a little lump in there that will make me ill so they are going to take it away and make me better again.'

'Oh,' he said, and was quiet for a minute. 'Do you mean an operation like Rhodri had on his back?'

'Yes, that's right, a similar thing but on my booby.'

25

'Hmm,' he said thoughtfully. 'Actually, I've got a bit of a bad back today,' and off he strolled towards Rhodri and Osh. So much for my angst in having to tell him. He is six – why would he be worried about it? I am glad that he is not older so that he can't understand what is happening.

August 3, Thursday

We have brought a mini DVD player with us and Osh's favourite film, *Winnie the Pooh*, and even though it is a beautiful film, it makes me feel incredibly sad. It starts off: '*Once upon the last day of a golden summer . . .* ' and I wonder if I will ever have a golden summer again after this one. And there is a song that Christopher Robin and Pooh sing which also makes me feel very sad, where Pooh is saying he is lost without Christopher Robin. And when he sings it, my heart feels as if it is breaking because I too feel so utterly, utterly lost and I wish someone would come and find me.

August 4, Friday

We leave Brittany today. Well, we almost didn't leave Brittany today as we were supposed to park the car on the other side of the barrier as it doesn't open until seven and we needed to leave at six thirty, so we had a blind panic and I suddenly realised what the French woman who came to make sure we had not trashed the caravan had been on about. I thought. I conducted that perfectly well with my few French phrases and a bit of give-us-a-clue, but what she was actually telling us was to park the car the other side of the barrier.

As luck would have it, I saw her cleaning the shower block and it is amazing how my command of the French language kicked in when we needed the barrier opened to enable us to get to the ferry port on time. It was all fine in the end and she opened the barrier and we got there with about half an hour to spare. To sum up my holiday, Brittany is sooo beautiful. I really want to come back here and if I ever had any money I would love to buy a little cottage on the sea front in Plouscat.

August 5, Saturday

Back in Wales, our holiday a distant memory now, I have washing and cleaning and an operation for a cancerous tumour to occupy my mind.

August 6, Sunday

I am packing for my trip to the hospital. Bizarrely, it feels as if I am going on a mini-break, which I jokingly said to Julia, my sister. The last time I packed a hospital bag was when I had Osh – and the time before that was when I had Elis. In my innocence, I really did think that it was going to be like a mini-break, until the reality of having a newborn baby who did nothing but cry 24/7 hit home. I realised that my days of mini-breaks were over, except that my lovely mother and father have made sure that I was able to have a few mini-breaks with Rhodri over the years. I have books and nice smellies and two pairs of my new pink gingham pyjamas and my little case and lots of healthy snacks. I seem to be forgetting the bit that I actually have to have the operation and that I have an illness that could kill me.

August 7, Monday

Rhodri's brother Owain and his girlfriend Eva get married a week Saturday. I am hoping that I am going to be well enough to go. I have a lovely dress which I got off eBay from China, don't you know, and it looks really lovely. We have a room booked for two nights in the St Bride's Hotel and if I can't go, Rhodri will take the boys on his own. That will be a bloody shock for him because I don't think he has ever had the both of them on his own overnight before.

I am in hospital tomorrow; you have to go a day before, to have various tests done – God knows what – so I'm all geared up to go. The children are up at my parents' farm so it was just me and Rhodri. I can't say he is the greatest help really. I just think he's a little boy sometimes and doesn't know what to say or do. We don't talk about anything.

August 11, Friday

I am home from hospital. On Tuesday morning I went to see the woman who did my biopsy at the Heath Hospital and she had to scan me and put a mark where the tumour was. She is this really great forthright Irishwoman. She was about an hour late and they said, 'Oh, you've missed your slot. Sorry, you could be waiting a long time,' but she arrives and turfs someone out of their room and says, 'Do you mind for five minutes, please?' and they leave like little sheep.

I asked her some questions about my tumour and she said, 'Now remind me how you came to us,' and I explained and she went, 'Oh yes, I remember you now. You were the person who came in and we thought nothing was wrong with you and then we found a tumour. Look,' she went on, 'you need to view this as a blip in your life, a year when you won't be feeling very well. Chemo isn't very

28

nice, but you will go through it and you will come out the other end. I say to women, "I'll see you in twenty years for a check-up" and they think I am joking but I really mean it.' And she asked me if I had children and she said, 'You are going to live a long life and look after your children.'

I said that no one had been so positive before and she replied, 'No, they won't tell you anything because they have to think in worst-case scenarios, but I'm telling you to see this as an inconvenience you have to go through.'

She also said, 'I see elderly patients who come in here when their partners have died – people they have spent fifty years of their lives with – and they come here and decide they've had enough and they want to die and they do because the mind is that powerful. So you need to be positive that you will get through it and have a long life.' She gave me a lifeline at that moment that I am clinging on to because I know they have to think of worst-case scenarios, but I don't want to be one; I want to look after my little boys until they can look after themselves.

Lovely Mr Monypenny came to see me just to reiterate what we had already discussed. He saw Dr Love's *Breast Book* and had a little smile to himself when I quoted something out of it, and said, 'The trouble with some books is that they give you too much information.' He is right about that; the book would also be very useful if the leg broke on your bed, as it is so thick and can be rather daunting. I deliberately put it in full view on my table so that the staff would realise I was practically as competent as them when it came to knowing about breast cancer. He said to me, 'Your lot (that's the BBC) are doing a programme on me and they are in here today.'

'God,' I said. 'Don't let them in here,' thinking that, worse than having a big lump cut out of your breast and arm, my colleagues seeing me without make-up would be terrible. I then had to answer hundreds of questions from other doctors (there is Mr Monypenny and there are other

29

doctors, that's how it is) and have blood tests – twice, because they lost the first lot. They ask you about your first period, breastfeeding, the age of having your first baby, the pill, alcohol consumption (I was slightly economical with the truth on that one, so have probably horribly skewed their statistics), who is looking after your children, who is looking after you, etc. I said to the doctor, who was very handsome but I felt I was old enough to be his mother, 'I'm ticking a lot of boxes,' and I asked him what they did with the info. He said that someone, somewhere does collate it to see if patterns emerge. They didn't ask, funnily enough, 'Are you riddled with self-doubt and anxiety?' They probably can't quantify that terribly well.

I also had to have an injection into my nipple. I wouldn't recommend this as a pastime, but I was very brave and did not cry. The nurse did warn me it would hurt and asked me to keep very still. I said I didn't think anything could be worse than childbirth and that most pain paled into insignificance in comparison. I now have a bright blue tit; at last I am a true 'Bluebird' which Rhodri, being the Cardiff City supporter he is, will no doubt appreciate. The dye in the needle finds the nodes under my arms and will show Mr Monypenny where they are when he cuts me open. Apparently the bright blue colour can take months to go.

Food was not good at the hospital even though I will really eat anything. The vegetarian option for dinner was quiche and chips; by this time I was so hungry, as my healthy snacks had gone, that I would have eaten a scabby-headed cat. I also had the nutritionalists' bible for breast cancer by my bed and wondered what Suzannah Olivier would have to say about quiche and chips and a mousse-type thing that defies description, to build you up the day before your operation. Oh well, at least the orange juice was healthy.

The ward was a bit of a shock. I dislike Llandough Hospital with a vengeance because the treatment I received when I had the children there was bloody horrendous. The maternity wards are very small but this ward had about twenty women on it and was a bit like a cattle market. The worst thing was that we were six breast cancer patients at the bottom of the ward and the rest of the ward were patients (mainly elderly) with things like bowel problems, or in the case of the nice lady next to me, a chest infection. She coughed all night and kept talking to me constantly and coughing over me. I know I have yet to qualify for my medical degree but it is surely a recipe for disaster that you keep surgery patients among other patients like that. No wonder Babs was out of hospital after two days with her drips hanging from her boobs because they had an infection on the ward – it must be a breeding ground for germs. The staff were lovely but horribly overworked, especially with so many elderly patients who had to buzz for everything.

I talked to Sandra, in the other bed next to me, who was having a mastectomy. She'd already had a lumpectomy but the cancer had spread to her nodes and they advised her to have it all off. I know that could be me in a couple of weeks if mine doesn't work out, but I AM thinking positively.

Rhodri came to see me the night before the op and we went for a walk. It was a sunny warm evening, the sun was setting and we looked at Cardiff below us and it was really beautiful – and for a minute I forgot why we were there and then I remembered and felt sad that this was happening to us.

The operation was surprisingly non-eventful. Yes, I felt like shit afterwards but not in pain from the operation itself. I just felt really drowsy but I almost like that state where you can't do anything, just lie there. How ironic that the only time I can sit down and not move is when I have been knocked out by a general anaesthetic. When I woke up on the Thursday morning I had no pain and I was talking to Sandra who had had the mastectomy and I thought, I've just had a lump out but she's just had her breast cut off, that must bloody well hurt, but she said it didn't. I said they must have given us really strong painkillers but when I asked, they'd only given us paracetamol! The body is remarkable; to have that done to you and not to feel pain is incredible. Don't get me wrong, if anyone came and poked me in the tit I might have had something to say about it, but it really is painless and I thought I would be in agony.

Elis has been up at my parents' farm for most of the week but Osh has come down for nursery. Sarah and Aidan are over from Ireland so they have been looking after him. Gwyneth over the road brought me some home-made Welsh cakes and I've had so many bouquets I've run out of vases.

Elis came home today but was very quiet. He seems to think that he can catch my illness because I have to stay off work, and you only stay off work or school if you have an illness and you don't want other people to catch it and get ill, so he didn't want to give me a kiss. I am not quite sure how you explain to a six year old that cancer isn't contagious. Of course, you must never use the 'C' word in case someone helpfully tells him what that is and at six you really don't need to know.

August 14, Monday

I haven't been doing much for the last few days, except resting really. I had some of my family down to see me – my mother and sisters over the weekend – but mainly I've been staying in and trying to rest. I still feel pain-free. Helen called and asked me how I was doing and said I might get spasms in my breast but they would pass very quickly, so there was no point taking any medication for them. However, I haven't had any. Perhaps the tumour was not very deep and there wasn't much tissue to cut through – and that is why it isn't painful.

The wedding is on now for the nineteenth, we are staying Friday and Saturday night so that should be good. I'm a bit apprehensive about it because even though Rhodri says he will look after the children I worry about them wandering off. So I am going on the proviso that I don't have to do anything other than turn up and eat. Owain has ordered non-alcoholic wine for me which he insists tastes just like the real thing. Elis has gone to stay with Sioned and Ali, Rhodri's aunt and uncle, for a week beforehand in Saundersfoot. They are having a break there before the wedding, so it's very quiet here and not much to do except eat chocolates and read magazines, at which I am becoming very adept.

August 18, Friday

We have arrived at the St Bride's Bay Hotel and it is really lovely; we have two rooms both with plasma tellies, a balcony (obviously an absolute no-go with the children); there are magnificent views over the bay. We had dinner with Sioned and Ali and picked Elis up. Elis has a three-piece suit for the wedding. He was insistent on having one and tried it on; his face was beaming and he said, 'I'm going to be the smartest man in the wedding.' The children loved the room although Elis tried to sneak in bed with us but we took him back.

August 19, Saturday

An eventful night and day. At five o'clock this morning the fire alarm went off. I used to be one of those people who didn't pay much attention to alarms and would dawdle out with my belongings until I was in an office in a factory once when a real explosion occurred and people were burned. Since then I've been bloody shit-hot at getting out when a fire alarm goes off.

Grabbing Osh, I gave him to Rhodri and snatched a blanket for Elis, as he never sleeps with any clothes on, and marched them all down the fire exit and outside. The people with children were the first out and like us they hadn't even stopped to pick anything up. Then out came everyone else, some quite hurriedly in their underwear or pyjamas. I was getting a bit concerned about Rhodri's parents, and then they arrived fully dressed with Rhodri's mother brushing her hair and carrying her handbag. The fire brigade turned up and although there was no sign of a real fire, we had to wait for an hour while the building was checked. Then they had to do a roll call of all the guests. Thank God it wasn't raining, otherwise I'd have been in that fire truck with Elis, who by this time had a duvet wrapped around him which the hotel manager had given him.

We eventually found out that the thermostat on the basement boiler wasn't working; it had overheated and set the alarms off. We were allowed to go back in our rooms but as we hadn't stopped to get the key, we had to wait outside for twenty minutes (we were the last room the manager opened) all practically asleep on the carpet by this time.

We got back into bed and I thought, This is it, they'll never sleep but they did, and we all slept in until about nine which was such a relief as I didn't think I could face the wedding on about five hours' sleep.

The wedding was lovely but for a horrible minute I thought that Owain wasn't going to go through with it. He came in and we were all assembled waiting for the bride to arrive and Owain was saying it was hot in there, which it was, but not that hot; the best man opened the windows, but Owain said he was still hot so the registrar got them to open some patio doors and fetched him a glass of water. I thought that was that, then the bride arrived looking

34

beautiful and radiant and, God, I'd marry her myself she was so stunning. So the registrar started her spiel (in two languages making it all very long) and Owain said he was hot again when it was coming up to vows time and had to stop and have a drink, then they went on a bit, then he had to stop again and take his jacket off and we were all looking at each other, both families doing polite smiles thinking, Oh, shit and I thought, Please God, don't have some dark secret now, Owain and all I could think about was would we still have the reception if they didn't go through with it, because I was starving. Then he just got hotter and hotter and then the registrar got him a seat and Eva was so attentive and caring and holding his hand, saying, 'Are you OK?' when, if it had been Rhodri, I'd be hitting him over the head and telling him to pull himself together.

So they eventually had to finish the ceremony with both of them sitting down, as it looked odd with just Owain sitting down. Eva eventually managed to get him to say all his vows, especially the 'I do' bit and he was hers. There was absolutely no way she was letting him get away – hot weather, shakes, sweats or dark secrets. It turned out that he hadn't gone to bed until two as he had been out with his mates, then he had to get up at five when the fire alarm went off. Then he couldn't go back to sleep so he had only had about three hours' sleep, which is not good, but there wasn't a dark secret in sight.

I forgot about the non-alcoholic wine and hit the real stuff and the children went to bed quite early. The telephones were a baby monitor so you could ring up from reception and hear them in the room – or not in our case. So we had a good drink and we went to bed about twelve.

August 20 Sunday

Woke up with a humungous headache. I have had to wear

35

sunglasses all morning indoors, even at breakfast. Owain said his friends thought I was very glamorous; they obviously thought I was trying to be enigmatic, not realising I was just horribly hungover. I said to Rhodri at the breakfast table, 'Thank God there wasn't a fire alarm last night. I would never have made it out of bed,' and he said, 'There was – you slept through it but it was the same problem, which they resolved, so everyone was allowed to go back to bed.' So much for the protective motherly instinct which seems to disappear once I've had a drink (or two)!

August 21, Monday

Back home. Operation hurting a little. I tried not to pick Osh up but it's easier said than done when you see a two year old about to do something he shouldn't. The kids were both so well-behaved at the wedding and Elis looked a picture in his suit although he only wore his shoes for the ceremony and was allowed to change into his trainers after I realised I'd bought his shoes a size too big. Elis was in Kids' Club this week which he loves and which means I can have a rest in the afternoons because he does really need entertaining – well, taken out to places.

I feel as if I'm neglecting them, which I know is silly, but two years ago I hadn't long had Osh so Elis was in nursery for most of the summer. I found it difficult to look after the two in the beginning, and last year we were having the house done and so the summer was a bit of a write-off. Then this year I was planning to take four weeks off work and have two for a holiday and another two at home going on day trips and doing mummy and son things, but that hasn't worked out. Now I'm home by myself and he's in Kids' club. I know he really likes it because he asks to go there, but I still feel guilty.

But I guess that's nothing to do with having an operation and being home alone: guilt is just a mother's lot in life.

August 22, Tuesday

Sarah's sister-in-law in Ireland, Fidelma, sent me some salt blessed by a priest to sprinkle on my food, and a prayer to recite over and over. Sarah is also getting the nuns to pray for me in the church and is having a mass said for me. On top of all that I have had a letter from a vicar who was on a programme that I was working on just before I left, who is also praying for me and my family. Another colleague from work – who is also a lay preacher – is saying prayers for me and the family. So, all in all, I am very well catered for in the praying department.

Rhodri – a strict non-believer – read the letter that Fidelma sent with her salt and I saw tears in his eyes. Hurrah! It's taken ten years, cancer and some holy salt, but at long last I've got him crying and expressing his emotions. Next time I'll just poke him in the eye. I get my results on Thursday and am counting down the days. I think it will be OK, but part of me doesn't want to think that, just in case it isn't and I have jinxed myself.

I guess if it isn't, I will have to have a mastectomy. It's ironic that my first reaction was to have a mastectomy, then after they mentioned that it is a bit of a drastic option, and not always necessary, you get used to the idea of saving your breasts. It's not the pain because, after having the lumpectomy, and after talking to Sandra about her mastectomy, and Babs, I know that it's not an unbearable pain, quite the opposite.

I did say that if I was going to have one off I would have them both off, which is part of the reason Babs had hers off, because I'm not exactly small in that department and you'd have to have one hell of a chicken fillet to match mine up.

We shall see.

August 23, Wednesday

Rhodri got the children up and out before I was up this morning. I must have drifted back off to sleep again, for when I woke up the sun was shining and I lay there for a few minutes coming to from sleep naturally – which hasn't really happened in the last seven years. I was lying there all cosy and relaxed and I thought to myself that something was wrong. I couldn't remember what and thought, Did I have a row with Rhodri last night and forget about it? and then I thought, No, that's not it, and I still lay there trying to think what could be wrong and then it hit me – Shit, I've got cancer.

For a few minutes there I had forgotten about the last few weeks and my diagnosis and my operation and all that stretches out in front of me, and I was the person I was before all this happened. I was a person without cancer living her life just like everyone else, and when I remembered that it wasn't so, a darkness came into my heart. I didn't cry and haven't cried really, not since this has happened, except one night when I was drunk with Rhodri in bed and on the holiday. I have been strong and held it together, as much for everyone else as myself, but there is a deep, deep sadness within me. It feels as if someone has left me without saying goodbye and I will never see them again. It is a physical pain in my heart, as if my heart is broken, and it is so deep, and so sad, that I'm not sure if it will ever go away.

August 24, Thursday

'Tomorrow's today' as Elis says when something exciting

is happening that he has had to wait for – except I'm not sure this constitutes excitement. I just want to go there, get my results, and get it over with. I am dressed in a black pencil skirt and a black three-quarter sleeve jumper and have fuck-off red lipstick on. I rarely wear bright red lipstick but when I do, it's a kind of 'here I am and you are not going to forget me' type of thing. I am also wearing my fuck-off red shoes (along the same lines as the lipstick).

Rhodri came with me for my results and I was glad, because when I went to get my results from the biopsy I couldn't take everything in; you need another pair of ears to remember things that are said.

Also, I tend to focus on all the negative things but Rhodri could put things in a bit more of a balanced way.

BBC Wales, my esteemed employer, are doing a programme about the Heath Hospital and coincidentally they are featuring the lovely Mr Monypenny, so every time I go to his clinic they are there with their bloody cameras, and the last thing I want is to be caught on camera by my colleagues. Also, Rhodri works for the BBC so it is slightly awkward when we are confronted by people whom we normally only see in a work setting at an intimate and, frankly, distressing, time in our lives. If I made this up, people wouldn't believe me. So we arrived and the cameras were rolling on the woman they were following and she happened to be sitting next to me, so I moved over behind a pillar because I didn't fancy exchanging pleasantries with the director and cameraman.

Then Mr Monypenny came out. 'Sorry,' he said, 'it's your lot again and you probably don't want to bump into them.' HE IS SO CONSIDERATE. So it's me and Rhodri and Mr Monypenny, and a breast nurse who I haven't seen before, in this little room and he says, 'The good news is that the nodes were clear.' This, he says, is 'the really good news' and he's smiling and I am smiling and I'm not sure about Rhodri because I'm looking at Mr Monypenny hanging on his every 'I am going to make you well again' words. Then he says, 'Unfortunately, we've got a bit of a problem.'

Other than a surgeon telling you you have cancer, the other thing you really don't want to hear coming out of his lips, when it is anything to do with you, is that there is a problem.

'*Houston, we have a problem.*' Didn't the shuttle explode after those words?

I don't want problems, I want it all to be OK and done and dusted so I can go home, but that isn't the case. You have to have clearance around your tumour of x amount, I can't remember what it is, but there has to be a clear margin so when they cut the tumour out they cut around it and take more than they need out, because there are microscopic cancer cells which they try to remove too.

Then they look at the extra tissue they've taken out and if they find that some of these cells are close to the margin they're not happy because they don't know how far they have spread out and they could form another tumour. I think that's how it all works, according to Susan Love and my interpretation of her book.

So the news is: I have microscopic cells that are close to the margins of the mass he removed and he wants to go in and have another go. My tumour is close to the breast wall, so he says there would be little point in giving me a mastectomy because he couldn't get any more clearance with a mastectomy than with a lumpectomy.

He said he could do it on 5 September and I could go home the same day, as long as someone could look after me. I was glad about that as I don't really want to go back in and stay, as I worry about MRSA and germs and flesh-eating bugs in that ward, with all those people who could be coughing over me, so in and out is fine with me.

I came out of his office and despite his lovely smiley reassuring face, I was in shock, as in all honesty, I hadn't really expected him to say that I would need another op. I kept focusing on the negative aspects and Rhodri would say, 'Yes, but he said it was good news that it hadn't spread,' and I would say, 'But they can't get clearance, and what if it spreads to my chest wall?' not really knowing what I was talking about, so it was like a conversation between someone with their glass half-full and someone with their glass half-empty.

I'm relieved of course that it hasn't spread, because I would then have to have had all my nodes out and probably a mastectomy as well, but I worry they won't get the clearance again and I'll end up having three operations in the space of a month and, as well as the physical aspect of it, it is so emotionally draining. We went for a coffee although I could have downed a gin and tonic. Rhodri kissed me and told me that when I walked into the hospital, I looked like a model, I was so beautiful, and I was glad I had my red lipstick on and my red shoes when I had bad news, because somehow they made it easier to face the world.

August 25, Friday

Rhodri is working away this weekend. Luckily he is around for the few days after my op so I don't need to get anyone down from my family to look after me. It is a Bank Holiday weekend this weekend, and Julia and Martin have taken Elis to Tenby with them and Lloyd, so it is just me and Osh.

August 26, Saturday

We are top of the league, we are top of the league. Rhodri is jubilant and rang me up to tell me this. Apparently Cardiff City is top of the league. I actually cannot stand football so am not entirely sure if including me in the 'we are top of the league chant' may not jinx the team completely. Football is the pain of my life for a number of reasons. 1) It is played entirely by men. 2) I know it is a cliché but the offside rule is unfathomable. 3) Rhodri is obsessed with it and is never in the house on a Saturday – well, every other Saturday – but the Saturdays he is here he has to listen to it or watch it. Our whole life is geared around this whole Cardiff City thing; we have had so many rows about it and thanks to his 'absolutely must attend at all costs' attitude, he has missed Elis's parties, me giving birth (well, post-giving birth), and our holidays have to be booked around it.

So I guess it's not Cardiff City I dislike *per se*, it's what they mean in my life. The day Osh was born, Rhodri, having already missed the birth and me being completely traumatised because I gave birth on my own without any midwives, went to see Cardiff City play. To say I was resentful and ever so slightly angry is a little bit of an understatement. I am getting a seething ball of anger in my stomach just writing this. It's such a man thing, I really don't get it at all. Although, saying that, Kerry is really into football and even understands the offside rule and she is not a man. Elis recently shouted during a match, 'Offside!' and Rhodri said, 'No, I don't think so.'

Paul in my office had gone to great pains to explain the offside rule to me in secret so I could miraculously comment on it, and I thought that I did actually understand it and I said to Elis, 'It's taken me nearly forty years to understand the offside rule and you are only six and get it,' and he said, 'No, I don't get it, I just shout it now and again.' And I thought. Bloody great! That's what I will do at around the point where offside usually occurs and see if any men in the room take me seriously – not that I particularly care about being taken seriously where football is concerned. It's just when Ian J comes over to watch the football with Rhodri, I really do not register with them in any way, shape or form as I am a woman and know nothing about football.

Football is the universal language of most men. Any man who is into football has instant 'man' currency. Women have it with other women who have children, but that of course is seen as fluffy and inconsequential because it is not football.

August 28, Monday

Went to stay with my mother and father for, as much as I crave some 'me' time, I don't want to be on my own. My mother and I took Osh for a walk along the canal and walked for miles. It was really lovely. I rarely get to spend time with my mother any more. I'm either dropping children off or picking them up and she does ring me EVERY DAY, so part of the problem is that I've nothing new to tell her. Plus she is always saying everything is going to be all right, and sometimes I just think, What if it *isn't* going to be all right? I am a mother myself so I can understand what she is going through, and if I was in the same position as her, I guess that I too would be telling myself and my child it was going to be all right as I would be too frightened to think of the consequences otherwise.

August 30, Wednesday

Elis is going up to Talybont to Rhodri's parents for a few days; he is coming back on Sunday. Rhodri is back today but gone again tomorrow and back Sunday. This time of the year is mad. Rhodri is never here for long, so juggling my life around cancer operations and looking after children isn't easy. I know it is Rhodri's job, but I doubt he has stopped to think about how I might be coping physically after my op and emotionally with having to have another one, *and* looking after the children and organising life as well.

He thinks all these things take care of themselves. I am sure he wants to be with his family, but there is a part of me that thinks buggering off, while your wife is diagnosed with cancer and having to look after two children and juggle arrangements for hospital appointments and operations while you stay in a nice hotel and go out for meals every night drinking wine and having adult conversations with people that don't involve cancer 24/7, cannot be that terrible. Fiddling while Rome burns springs to mind – him, that is, not me. I don't have time to fiddle.

September 1, Friday

Calm calm calm. Deep breaths. Elis is still at Rhodri's parents' and Osh is in the crèche so I have a bit of head space. I guess I shouldn't complain; some women don't have the luxury of a day or two to themselves. I still don't seem to have time to sit down much: I'm always doing something, like sorting Osh's clothes out or tidying cupboards in Elis's bedroom, anything rather than sit down and contemplate what is really going on in my life and my mind.

I know that after my second op, my chemotherapy will start a few weeks later, and I haven't got my head around that and what it means. I have of course consulted Susan Love on this and I know it affects different women in different ways; I just wish I knew what my way was and if it is as bad as people say it is.

My mother keeps telling me about all the people she knows who have had chemotherapy OR whose daughters/aunties/sisters/cousins have had it. There is always someone, it seems, every day whom my mother has met who has a story to tell which she has to relay back to me in intricate detail. I know my mother is trying to be positive, BUT I really don't want to know about other people at the moment; it's enough of a head-fuck coming to terms with it all myself.

Babs introduced me to a woman called Beth who has breast cancer; she is younger than me by about two years and also has two young children. She has had a mastectomy and is going through chemotherapy.

Helen the breast nurse had told me that she had one patient who couldn't get out of bed with her chemo but that was quite unusual; most women feel unwell and sick but can go about doing their daily tasks.

Beth, it transpires after chatting with her for a while, is Helen's patient who cannot get out of bed. After she has had her chemotherapy she is in bed for four days and cannot move. She said, 'I literally cannot open my eyes and get out of bed.' This is not really what I wanted to hear but I guess I have to put plans in place (because no one else will unless I do) in case this happens.

I've relayed this information to my mother and sisters and they of course have agreed to have the children or come down and stay when I have the chemo or whenever I need them. I don't know what I would do without them; I know that they will be there for me and it makes this whole bloody mess so much easier to bear.

September 4, Monday

Rhodri is away doing the Proms, my second op is tomorrow, so consequently I haven't had time to brood about it too much. Osh is up at my mother's for a few days and Elis is starting back to school on Wednesday, so he has to be in Cardiff on Tuesday night. It has sort of arrived really. I have packed a bag just in case I need to stay in, but am hoping it will be fairly routine and I will be in and out. In a way I just want to get it over with so that I can get on with the chemotherapy; perverse as that may sound, the sooner that is over with, the better, I think.

I have been on the internet and ordered some turbans, hats and scarves in case I feel the need to wear them at any time. The site sells hats for chemotherapy. However, Kylie managed to look pretty gorgeous in her scarves so you never know, I might pull it off. I am also getting oversized glasses à la Kylie so if my eyelashes and eyebrows fall out, then they will be covered by even cooler sunglasses. The look I am aiming for is a frail vision of loveliness, although it will probably be more akin to a dodgy shoplifter.

Oooh, they do a hat called the 'muff' hat; I will get Rhodri one of those for Christmas. They also have a cancer 'gifts' section – trust the bloody Americans to come up with that one. They are kitsch teddies with verses on them about love and friendship. I shouldn't scoff, I know. They also have a section for children's wigs which makes you stop laughing at all this and makes your heart break.

September 7, Thursday

I had my operation on Tuesday. Rhodri and I had a terrible row beforehand. He took me to the hospital and I was a little stressed, understandably I might add, and as we got in the car, I said, 'I haven't got any money or anything now as I don't want to leave any valuables in my locker,' and he said, 'Fine, don't worry about it.'

So we drove there, and when we got to the car park, he said 'Have you got any money? I haven't brought any,' and I said no, I didn't, and that I had told him so.

46

So he said he didn't have any change to put in the meter to park the car, but, 'Well, never mind – I'll just drop you off at the entrance.'

I couldn't believe it. I said, 'What do you mean? I'm going into hospital for a fucking operation for cancer and you want to drop me off at the front door?' and he said, 'No, I don't *want* to. I just said that because I felt stupid because I didn't bring any money,' and I was furious. I could have happily stabbed him at this point.

So I went on about how this was about more than the money: it was about his complete inability to have any understanding as to what the hell I might be going through, and as I got my stuff out of the boot, I noticed some money in there and I couldn't have cared less if he came in with me or not because I didn't even want to look at him.

So he put the money in the meter and followed me in, carrying my bag. I was furious and I started to cry in the stairwell on the way up and he was saying how terribly sorry he was and he did understand what I was going through so I forgave him, but only because I didn't want any bad karma going into my operation, which was what he should be bloody well thinking as I am the one about to go under the surgeon's knife once again.

The ward I was originally on was full so I got my own private room – hurrah! It was bliss, although I did think that someone could come in and murder me and no one would know, it was so quiet in there. I read my book, watched a bit of TV and generally relaxed, so by the time my op came I was a picture of serenity; a far cry from when I had arrived.

A porter took me down, there was a bit of a delay in the pre-op room and I was chatting to him and one of the nurses about life, the universe, where we lived, how many children we had, when Mr Monypenny came in, he smiled beatifically, said, 'Hello,' then started looking at my notes.

I said, a little anxiously, 'Have you forgotten what you

are doing?' and he smiled again and said, 'No, I'm just reminding myself how much breast tissue I have left to cut away.' I said, 'Oh, OK,' thinking he sees bloody hundreds of women, of course he looks at their notes before operating on them.

Then he said, 'Your lot are here again. They filmed me doing an operation this morning. I checked to see if you were on the ward because they were filming there, but you were in a side ward, otherwise you could have moved'.

As he was talking, I saw, over his shoulder, the film crew with their bloody cameras. I half-expected my work colleagues to pop up and say, 'Candid camera!'

So he left and the porter said to me, 'That man is one of the best in the country, you know, not just Cardiff,' and I thought, Yes I do know and thank God for that.

They wheeled me down to pre-op and Mr Monypenny was there again and I said to the anaesthetist, 'Tell me when you are going to put that needle in because I want to be thinking happy thoughts.' I wanted to think about my children walking through long grass, for some reason. I asked Mr Monypenny how the filming was going and he chatted to me about it as if we were having a cup of tea, not like someone who was about to take another chunk out of my breast. It was all very civilised, if a little bizarre.

I came around after the op and my breast was very painful, much more so than the first time around. I guess that is where the saying 'opening old wounds' comes from. So I had loads of morphine and spent the rest of the day, until Rhodri came, in a bit of a morphine haze, although I did manage to polish off a three-course lunch without any problems. The next day I was supposed to have an appointment with Rosie, an acupuncturist, who was recommended to me by Richard E, who has been such a great help with books and advice. He says cancer is about the immune system and acupuncture helps the immune system. I will give it a go soon, but I got Rhodri to cancel it, as the thought of anyone sticking another needle in me is a bit to much too bear at the moment. I get my results on Thursday so I don't have long to wait.

September 10, Sunday

I have spent the weekend pottering, which is something I do exceptionally well. With two children, pottering is turned into an art form; just as one thing is picked up, another goes down and so the cycle goes on and on, so instead of calling it cleaning, women where I come from tend to call it pottering, to mask the mundane banality of it all. I am still taking it easy because that second op knocked me for six. I just hope that they have it all this time, because if they don't I will have to go and have a mastectomy. To have gone through two operations only to be told I have to have a third would, I think, make me feel a bit let down.

September 11, Monday

My period has started today. Thank God it didn't come when I was having my ops. In Susan Love's book there is supposed to be an optimum time in your menstrual cycle for operating for breast cancer. Susan Love works in an American system and mentions asking to reschedule your operation to fit in with your menstrual cycle. I don't really have this luxury, but coincidentally, both operations did fall into this timeframe so I am pleased about that.

I am trying to find out as much as I can, being a fully qualified Google doctor, but some of the sites are downright scary, and statistics on survival are all five and ten years and I think, Shit I was hoping for a bit more than that.

My mother (yet again and I try not to listen) was telling me about a woman who had breast cancer when she was forty and she is in her late sixties now and I said, 'Great, give me twenty years, I would be very happy.' She says, 'She has had more than twenty years, Shelley, so don't go worrying about it.'

I don't think people can fully understand just how much you will, of course, worry about it – to the point that it can make you feel physically sick. It is all I think about, my life expectancy: will I be able to get rid of this, will they be able to remove it all? So I feel like screaming at anyone who tells me not to worry, it will be OK, because the truth is, no one – not me, not my mother, not the woman who has lived more than twenty years, and not even my surgeon – knows if I will be OK. Only time will be able to reveal that little secret.

September 12, Tuesday

I have again decided to learn Welsh. Rhodri is a first-language Welsh speaker, Elis is fully bilingual and Osh can say a few words and Rhodri always speaks to him in Welsh so there's this little clique in our house of three men all babbling away in Welsh and then there's me. I can *deall* (understand) a lot of Welsh but don't really speak any, so I need to start from scratch. I feel I need to structure my time in some way over the next few months and this is a good opportunity to do it, when I don't have the constraints of work. It will take my mind off my illness. Am I ill? I don't feel ill. I'm not quite sure how to describe what I am. I was fine until they found my tumour-type thing. I am embracing Suzannah Olivier's book on nutrition and am basically having a vegetarian diet. My sister looked at it and said she thought it was difficult to follow but as I was a vegetarian for eleven years before I met Rhodri I find it easy, and I love salads and pulses so it's not a big deal.

I'm also the proud owner of the Champion Juicer and am juicing for Britain. I will be the purest woman in Llandaf and Llandaf has some very pure people in it, being a theological city. Basically fat and dairy are a no-no, as is red meat. Chicken is fine in moderation but I must try to stick to vegetarian with chicken a few nights and the occasional Sunday roast.

As Suzannah Olivier says, 'you have to let your hair down now and again.' While you still have it, I thought, when I read it. Fish is also good but I am not really a big fish eater so I find that quite difficult, but am trying smoked, peppered mackerel which I can just about eat if I take the shiny skin off the back.

I am continuing with my supplements and the man-boy in the healthfood shop (who is bloody gorgeous) is *very* knowledgeable about supplements and breast cancer. The fact that I could say 'breast cancer' to him and he didn't wither away is one thing, and another is that he actually has some knowledge – in fact he almost quoted Suzannah Olivier's list verbatim, such a God of Supplements is he.

September 13, Wednesday

We have just returned from the hospital en famille. Osian ate one of the hawthorn berries which are littered around the garden. His brother has managed to survive six years without so much as looking at a berry because I drummed it into his head from a foetus that berries were dangerous and you would die if you ate one, while simultaneously trailing my fingers across my throat as if someone were cutting it with a knife. I somehow forgot to do this with his younger brother (you are ALWAYS more relaxed with the second

51

one) so Osh sat on the grass chomping away while I unloaded the dishwasher and his father played football with Elis. After Rhodri had discovered him eating them and got him to clear his mouth he thought he had probably only swallowed one. I immediately rang the NHS helpline who took an age to answer, then set about asking me unanswerable questions: was he complaining that his throat was constricting? Uh hello – he's two, and have you ever tried to open the mouth of a two year old, when he didn't want you to, to assess if his throat was constricting? Was he complaining of an upset stomach or any stomach cramps? He can't speak yet and when he does it's a mixture of two languages, so it's difficult to know what he is saying at the best of times. Fine, they would call me back within the next four hours. So I did my usual self-assessment on Dr Google, and the first entry under the search of *Berries, hawthorn and poisonous* was *Hawthorn berries are VERY POISONOUS* – so upped the family and went to Casualty. Elis, who has had the drummed-in berry phobia for the last six years, kept asking if Osian was going to die. At which point I replied with my philosophical cancer head, 'We are all going to die but it's not Osian's day today.'

On arrival at Casualty, the so-called casualty ran up and down the corridors shouting, 'Clown!' at the top of his voice to the clowns on the walls. By the time we got to see a doctor it was clear that, after almost an hour, he was not going to keel over, and the doctor's toxicity database, which he showed me (clearly recognising my medical stature) said that in small doses hawthorn berries would not cause much harm apart from an upset stomach. I should give the patient milk, which I had already done, – having had experience of this when he sucked some Domestos.

'We're a twenty-four-hour service, so if you are worried, bring him back,' he said. Ah, the good old NHS, I do love them.

Arriving back home, it was straight to bed for both of

them – no bath, no cleaning of teeth, just a story for Elis from Rhodri while I tucked Osian up. Osh snuggled under his new duvet and still looked like a small baby despite being nearly two and a half and I looked down at him and my heart flipped over because I loved him so much it hurt a little bit.

I was about to kiss Elis good night when I discovered another medical emergency: one of his fish was floating on top of the water on its side, barely alive. I fished him out and put him in a bowl with a bit of salt in it – a trick I learnt off my dad. It worked with him before when he was ill (on the fish, that is, not my dad). Then, I took the other one out and put him in a separate bowl so he was out of the contaminated water – it was too late at night by this time to clean the tank. I put some thoroughly washed sea shells and a fossil in the tank the other day so they could have something to swim around and I wonder if there was something on them that poisoned the tank. Perversely, I could be a poisoner. Fingers crossed he'll pull through; let's hope it's not his day today.

My test results come through tomorrow. A week ago it seemed like a lifetime, this morning I thought Thursday was days away, then I realised it's tomorrow. I had planned a quiet evening of rest and contemplation and a bit of Welsh homework. Now I have an hour and a half to fit in Welsh homework, Tuesday's episode of *Lost* and a bit of *Heat* magazine all before bedtime. Ho hum. Better have one more look at the little darlings and the family pets (pet?). What is it they say? 'Life is what happens when you are making other plans.' That was certainly true tonight.

September 14, Thursday

Oooh ooh ooh good news! Good news! More good news! Wonderful, life-saving, fantastic Mr Monypenny has got clearance around my tumour and is 'very happy' with it. What a bloody relief. No more surgery, hurrah! Straight on to chemotherapy; do not pass Go, do not collect £200. I'm 'on the good side of bad' he says, about 75 per cent (not quite sure of what, maths never being one of my strengths) but 75 per cent sounds good. I'll take that, thank you very much, Mr Monypenny. I think it probably refers to the cancer returning to the same spot. I'll ask the double-barrelled oncologist when I see him – whom I will also fall in love with, according to Beth. With chemo and radiotherapy and Tamoxifen, the odds go higher and higher, but I'll probably be glowing in the dark after all that toxicity. Who cares? Bring it on.

After skilfully avoiding the film crew for two months, there they were in the waiting room again, following the lady sitting behind me. Both Rhodri and I took a sudden interest in the posters on the wall as Rhodri had recently worked with the cameraman and we weren't in the mood for chit chat about breast cancer over a skinny latte at that point in time.

We moved to the 'before you have breast cancer and are being screened' part of the waiting room where the women look like frightened bunnies, as opposed to the 'we've got breast cancer' part of the room, where they look slightly less anxious – having had the bad news – and slightly more eager to get in there and find out what the prognosis is. Anyway, Mr Monypenny came over to the 'before side' to talk to us so we didn't bump into 'my lot' as he refers to them.

I thanked him VERY much when I left and shook his hand, as did Rhodri. I probably won't see him again, and parting is such sweet sorrow. Not seeing him again is, of course, a good thing, a great thing, as I wouldn't want the breast tumour to return BUT if it did, I would definitely want to see him again.

Suddenly, with the shake of a hand, the man who has

saved my life is gone, on to the next patient who is lucky enough to have him as his or her surgeon. However, thanks to the good ol' BBC, I'll be able to see him on the telly programme, whereupon I can rewind, fast forward and pause him, in all his loveliness, to my heart's content.

The other good news is that Fishy the goldfish survived the night, although we are not out of the woods yet. He is buoyant and blinking and opening and closing his mouth regularly (very important vital signs in a fish – God, I'm a qualified vet now as well as a qualified breast surgeon and oncologist) as opposed to floating with a fixed stare, and he has eaten food. I poked him and he didn't dart around the bowl but did move a bit. He also looks as if he has a small tumour on his head – nothing too big – and I had another fish which lived for ten years with a tumour on its head. My God, I've got something in common with one of the family pets! I am to Fishy what Mr Monypenny is to me – a lifesaver – although I may possibly be the one who caused his near death-like state in the first place, with the fossil or shells that were in the tank. I have the power of life and death in my hands over two orange and silver bodies – bloody hell, what a responsibility.

Anyway, after my long lunch with Babs, I will thoroughly clean out the tank, removing the offending shells and fossil, and put Rods back in. Fishy will have to remain in his private ward under strict observation until he is deemed fit enough to return to the tank without fear of killing Rods off. I think I might pop into the pet shop and buy some fish-friendly tank adornments as a get-well present.

I don't know if it is the fact that my cancerous tumour is gone, but I feel very Zen about the world. Am thinking of becoming a Buddhist, and will do a bit of Googling on that when I get a minute. The only thing is I can't kill anything if I am a Buddhist, and I'm not sure I can uphold that ideal if one of those huntsman spiders is in the same room as me as it was the other night (the size of my hand), when I don't have Rhodri to come between me, it, an encyclopaedia and sudden death.

God I could come back as one of those – oooh, just had a slight inkling as what it must be like to be a huntsman spider with everyone on the planet (excluding David Attenborough and presumably his film crew who couldn't do that if they were afraid of creepy crawlies and Buddhists other than myself) can't stand the sight of you. I want to apologise on record now to any spiders I might have inadvertently squashed with an encyclopaedia in the past and, Lord Buddha, if you are reading this, could I please come back as a sleek, black (so my colour) pampered cat with a diamanté collar – and loads of road sense? But not just yet. Can I get over my cancer first and have at least twenty years while my children grow up? Thanks, Buddha.

September 15, Friday

Rhodri is back in our bed again after nine days. Firstly, it was because I was not compos mentis after the drugs, then he had 'man's flu'. In fairness he did have a bad cold but I had little sympathy for him. I am paranoid about germs as I am trying to ensure my immunity is strong before I start the chemo, which will wipe it all out anyway. So there was another five days because of man flu until there was not so much as a sniff out of him. He was banished to the Bob the Builder duvet section of Elis's bunk beds. God, it's been bliss having a king-size bed to myself. We are not really meant to sleep together – not just me and Rhodri, I mean, but everybody. There's always one who fidgets (Rhodri), one who needs stillness (me), one who is always hot (Rhodri) and one who is always cold (me). Who said opposites attract?

I keep meaning to buy one of those two-singles-but-a

double beds so you are together apart, but I never seem to have any 'spare' money to do that. God, do people REALLY have spare money? How much money do you have to be earning before you have spare money? It must be a shedload because we never have any money, ever, and I wouldn't say we have a particularly extravagant lifestyle. I think eBay may have something to do with it though. I don't want to even think about credit cards at the moment: moneysaver.com is my lifesaver.com.

Lovely Martin Lewis really has saved me a fortune with his savvy advice and boy-next-door good looks, but even he can't magic away my humungous credit card bills. But anyway I have bigger things to think about now than being bogged down by the trivia of things, like debt. I am in a higher spiritual place at the moment and when I get back to reality I can think long and hard about another 'consolidation', as it is so helpfully called.

Just to be sure, I have poked a sleeping Rhodri in the shoulder to ask him to swear on Osian's life that he doesn't have any hidden credit cards. He does that – he gets credit cards and hides them, but of course he is too stupid, OK, I hate that word, no, I can't think of another suitable word, too *stupid*, to hide the bills from me or in fact the actual credit card. This usually ends in a blazing row with me passing him some scissors and him cutting it up in front of me.

He complained that I had woken him up – hmm, the vast expanse of the king-size bed gets smaller and smaller when you have a grizzly bear in it. Then within two minutes he was asleep again – how can he do that? It takes me ages to get to sleep. It's not fair. Anyone who can go to sleep that quickly HAS to be a self-centred individual, otherwise they would be thinking about umpteen other things other than being happy and content with their wonderful selves.

Now, thinking about money, *I* can't get to sleep. Richard E, with whom Rhodri has been working, brought me three books which are by the side of my bed, and one especially, *The Drama of Being a Child*, is beckoning to me. I think it's a little too much to bear this week, as looking after my own children is enough of a drama in itself at the moment. I will endeavour to start it next week. I'll just read a little bit of *Heat* tonight. Sadly, even the exploits of ex-*Big Brother* housemates can't rest my mind. I think the underlying crux of my restlessness is a dawning realisation that with all that's happened over the last day, seeing Mr Monypenny and talking about statistics, for once, throughout this whole bloody process, I have allowed myself the indulgence of thinking that I am not going to die – I mean not going to die *now* – never mind in the bloody future when I'm old and grey (although I will of course never allow myself to go grey).

I WANT TO LIVE NOW OK. I DON'T WANT TO BLOODY WELL DIE, FOR MY CHILDREN, FOR MY HUSBAND, FOR MY FAMILY AND FRIENDS, AND MOST OF ALL, YES MOST OF ALL, FOR ME. I don't want to die and I don't want to tell people that because they are all so positive and upbeat because I am too; but when push comes to shove, when all's said and done, I want to live. I want to live to a ripe old age and go on Saga holidays with Rhodri and have a flat in Tenby and walk my dog, if Rhodri will ever let me have one, on the beach and spoil my grandchildren, and in order to do all those things I'm going to have to live a long time. So God, Buddha, Mohammed or any other deities who may or may not be listening, give me a go, eh? I'm quite a nice person, really. I am a good mother, sometimes a good wife. I have my moments, and I could try harder and I will. That I promise you.

September 16, Saturday

Tonight my mother and father are looking after the children

58

and we are going out with Ian J. Everyone keeps saying to crack open a bottle to celebrate the news that I don't need more surgery. Everyone is ecstatically happy, which is lovely to hear, but I'm still erring on the side of caution. Why? I still have a niggle and the last time I had that niggle I had cancer. Now I'm thinking about God and warnings from above to change my lifestyle and sort myself out. OK, if You are there and You are reading my diary, I'm trying my best, really I am. I'm trying not to drink so much and doing really well with that, God.

I'll be a better wife and a better mother, and I will be patient with my children, and I will learn to say no and I will try my very best to do something in the community, and I will love animals and try not to kill spiders and not think unkind thoughts about people I may or may not be jealous of. I'll do all of those things and more, but please let me live a long life, please please please let me bring up my own children. That's all I want, for them to be well-rounded, loved and cherished human beings. And their mummy's heart breaks every time she thinks about them having to grow up without her.

Not that Rhodri wouldn't do a sterling job. How could I possibly wish for a better father? He is so incredible with them and they wouldn't have to grow up with a mother who was so totally paranoid about them hurting themselves or getting knocked over or falling from trees that it made her heart miss a beat with worry sometimes. Is it normal to fear all of the time that something is going to happen to them? Now that something has happened to me, I have to learn how to be less paranoid about them.

September 17, Sunday

I was very sensible last night, which Ian J commented on. Tried to stay on the water but also had a few glasses of wine. It's odd, but when the children are here all I want is a bit of peace, and now they are not here, all I do is think about getting them back again.

I thought about writing a letter when I was diagnosed: a 'mummy loves you more than life itself' letter, but the practicality of it all meant that I wouldn't need to do it in the first week, that I would at least see a few more months out before I was at the letter-writing stage. As time has progressed and each stage has passed, I still think about that letter a lot, but what I would write in it in has changed beyond recognition. Maybe this period of reflection has given me an inner strength and the inner peace that I am, I think, beginning to feel. Please, let it be real. I want to feel calm like this all of the time.

No, the letters would be different to the ones that I started penning in my head in July. To my children they would be letters about the wonderful memories of them as babies and growing up, and the funny things they have said which you forget so easily, but think you will remember for ever, but mainly they will be about my love for them. How you can describe that in a letter is the question – there is a pain in my heart as I write this – but to remind them how wonderful they are, how they came into the world with so much love, and what they can be in life.

The biggest change has come in the letter I would write to Rhodri. It started off as a manual of all the things he should and shouldn't do; how I thought this should be done with them, and that should be done with them, things not to forget like sun cream and gym bags and reminding him to tell them he loved them and to hold them. But then I thought that I actually have no right to tell him how to bring up our children. If I were not here, that is for him to decide, and as for reminding him to tell them he loves them and to hold them, his love for them is evident in every action he does for them and with them. I would thank him for our life together, 'sometimes good, sometimes bad, sometimes bloody awful, sometimes bloody amazing', much like everyone else, really, and for making me a whole person and for loving me and putting up with me and to never ever ever mix colours and whites in the washing machine. Dear God, if You are listening, I would settle for a minimum of twenty years – that would be top banana, really it would. My children would be all grown up and hopefully with some idea of how to fend for themselves. They will not go into the world being a rod for another woman's back, the house will be paid for, and even Rhodri could go off and find himself a lovely young wife who isn't afraid of spiders, who would love to go to South Africa without worrying about being mugged, and who takes an interest in world politics and knows what the hell is going on with the Israelis and the other bunch. A wife who already speaks Welsh and loathes the Labour Party – he would be in his element for sure.

I'm 75 per cent and rising with every toxic cocktail on offer, so I know I should be REALLY happy too. I'm on the good side of bad. I am on the good side of bad, I am on the good side of bad.

September 18, Monday

Hmm, just had a thought about Rhodri's new 'in the event of my death' (ITEOMD) wife. Was cleaning the kitchen floor, which incidentally was minging – thank God for slate, it's a great hider of dirt. I do seem to have eureka moments while doing the housework. If I didn't have to worry about things like French doors being smear-free or getting quotes for new windows and children's gym bags, I too could sit down at the internet and read papers and find out about the Palestinians and the other lot.

So although Rhodri's new (ITEOMD) wife might come to the relationship well versed in world affairs, she too would have to take up the smear-free French windows gauntlet, wouldn't she? Then she wouldn't have a bloody clue either about what was going on in the world because she would be too knackered on a daily basis to bloody well care – except, of course, on a human level of caring that people are living in fear and getting hurt kind of way. By *Newsnight* time – see? I don't even know what time that is on, and I have sat in on TV scheduling meetings for the last four years – I want to do nothing more exerting than read about ex-*Big Brother* housemates and their exploits in *Heat* magazine.

Unless she didn't care about them of course – the windows, that is, not people living in fear of their lives on a daily basis. BUT oh shit, I've just thought he could meet her in work and she could be a bloody BBC journalist, then her job would be to know those things on a daily basis. Ah, but then Rhodri would feel threatened by her superior knowledge of world affairs or he could be in awe of her and that would make her more attractive – bugger bugger bugger. Must start telling him how crazy and mad journalists are to put him off them.

September 19, Tuesday

Went to see the acupuncturist today, Rosie, who is very nice and very calm. The first session is about two hours long and is like a counselling session. She sits you down and asks you why you came and then asks other questions about your life and your work and your relationships. I think it is probably the first time in my entire life that I have said some of the things I have said to anyone in such a coherent way.

The questions kept coming back to me and Rhodri and our relationship, and we ended up mainly talking about that, not my illness. She says she needs to understand where the illness might be coming from. So I say that I am controlling and bossy and that he is emotionally immature and quite selfish. It was very enlightening, as I know I'm quite controlling but I've never seen it as a major problem, and usually make light of it, saying, 'I'm a control freak,' but I *am* a control freak and that does manifest itself in a lot of anxiety in my life, especially with the children. I feel that I have to control them because if they listen to me and do exactly as I say, then they can't hurt themselves. Not sure that works with Rhodri but I think I control Rhodri because I cannot live with a man who thinks he could control me. My father was very paternalistic to us as children and I never want to feel like that again. Here I am subjecting my own children to my control and it's taken an acupuncturist to show me.

September 21, Thursday

Oh my God, have been reading *The Drama of Being a Child* and there is synchronicity in this world because it is all about . . . controlling our children. I am reading on and resolving to be a less controlling, more giving and accepting mummy. I am, I am, I am. I have discussed my Rosie conversations with Rhodri and told him I thought we needed to go to a counsellor; he squirmed and wriggled like a worm but said yes only because I have cancer. Told Rosie this and she thought it was very positive.

September 22, Friday

Rhodri has been in Leeds for a week doing a piano competition. Life has been busy with two wee ones to look after on my own – although, of course, staying at home with only Welsh class and lunching with friends to keep me occupied (oh, and obsessively tidying the house) and someone else actually looking after my children between the hours of 9 and 5 is not exactly challenging.

I am feeling rather guilty about staying at home as I'm not ill now I've got over my operations, so I'm doing housey things like making chilli and shepherd's pie for my family. I feel like a real homemaker, mother and wife – the epitome of the 1950s housewife.

The truth is, I really like being at home. I'd rather be making shepherd's pie and picking my children up early and sitting down and helping them with their spelling or their maths rather than relying on overworked teachers to do everything. If someone had told me two years ago that I would have written that, I would never have believed them. I don't know where this person has come from, but I just want to be with my children and at home.

If I could stay home all the time, I wouldn't get fat and I wouldn't watch daytime TV. I would just do my Welsh, potter in the garden, potter in the house, meet my friends, pick blackberries, find conkers with my children, have other people's children over to play – and I've described my perfect existence.

If I didn't have to work, I'd have Osh at home for most of the week and just be a cooking, cleaning, lunching yummy (of course) mummy – except we need the money. The reason I have nice 'things' and a nice house and never think too much about credit card consolidation and children's shoes is because I go out to work and work pays me money and money buys me stuff. I must remember to look up the Buddhist thing because I think Buddhist philosophy mentions stuff and ownership. Must do that, it's not as if I haven't got any time on my hands to be doing this or reading Richard E's books. I have also banned myself from eBay for the time being. I actually had to go to town to drop the car off in the garage this morning and realised you can get great bargains there too – that was a bit dangerous. I never go into town because it's too much hassle as I usually have at least one child with me. I will be 'popping' into town again soon to get the bumper fixed on the car where I went into the back of a Jaguar – yes, a bloody Jaguar – a new one as well. It was my fault – she stopped, I didn't, and she was so lovely about it all, saying, 'Never mind. At least you didn't have your children in the car,' pointing at the boys' car seats. Ah, women are so even-tempered and practical. I bet if it was a bloke he'd have been calling me all the names under the sun, children's car seats or no children's car seats.

September 24, Sunday

Joanne came over to stay this weekend with Megan (four), and Julia was moving up to Mum's. She has sold her house so is staying there while she finds a suitable house or plot to build on so we had Lloyd (four) with us. Not a bad ratio, two adults to four children under seven. We drank two bottles of wine on Saturday night. TOP TIP – looking after four small children and drinking a bottle of wine DO NOT GO TOGETHER.

It is not as if this is the first time I have done this and doubtless not the last either, but will I ever learn? I made Joanne vegetarian fajitas with Quorn which she raved about; they were very nice but after that much wine and not eating until nine o'clock, anything would have been wonderful.

We didn't go to bed until late and we had a really nice time talking about life, the world and the universe. Why is it whenever I'm looking after a group of children I stupidly think they won't wake up until late because they went to bed late? Life doesn't work like that; they were all up by seven. So we took the only course of action open to two hungover adults: we let them play mindless games on the

Playstation, had children's TV on in two rooms, fed them chips and rubbish, let them trash the house and then took them to the park to wear them all out.

September 25, Monday

Rhodri came back from Leeds – was glad to see him for about half an hour then he started asking me banal questions which got my blood boiling, like why was I recording children's films on Sky Plus and why was I doing this and why was I doing that. After a week on my own without anyone to question me or upset my routine, and spending quality time with the children and Sky Plussing to my heart's content, it gets on my nerves. If we were fabulously wealthy we could have separate wings of the house and come together for food, sex and other stuff that doesn't spring to mind – um, like children things. We tend to watch different programmes, apart from one, so we don't even really watch the telly together.

I bet if we had separate wings he'd be pestering me in my wing for stuff (probably as a precursor to getting his leg over) but at last those banal conversations that drive me mad would mostly be dispensed with. I wonder if Madonna and what's-his-name do that?

It would make for a bloody happy marriage, I'd say. Anyway, a bit later on he was sat in the living room and I went in and paused the Champion's League because I wanted to have a cancer conversation with Rhodri and thought that maybe, just maybe, he was growing up a bit. I was crossing my fingers and toes in anticipation.

I said that Jane had dropped Lloyd off with Julia and she asked me twice how I was after I had asked her how she was, as she is very pregnant.

I couldn't understand why she asked me pointedly twice how I was – then it clicked. Shit, I've got cancer – or I *had* cancer, depending on how you look at it – and I'd forgotten. So I told Rhodri that I had forgotten I had cancer and that since seeing Mr Monypenny I was feeling that it was all OK now. I was going to live and I was seeing the chemo- and radiotherapy as minor blips to get over and I would live a long life and I thought I'd become complacent that this was it; I was cured and I felt guilty about feeling that I was cured and had not dared to speak of it before, and now I had gone from one extreme to another.

Firstly I spent the best part of two months obsessing that I might die or certainly not live long, and now I have become so complacent that I had actually forgotten about it when Jane asked me about it. I just feel a fraud that I had a cancerous breast tumour and had two ops which didn't really hurt that much and didn't really make me ill, and that I was enjoying the time I spent at home and felt guilty about enjoying it – and even though I know chemotherapy isn't going to be nice, it's short term and I can deal with it and then I will have radiotherapy and life will go back to normal. Will it, will it? Am I mad? Am I deluded? Am I naïve? Am I just fooling myself into believing that this is it – that I'm OK and something will happen to wipe the supercilious smile off my face?

Rhodri, who did not object to the pausing of the Champions League (the beauty of Sky Plus), said,' You've had a life-threatening illness; you are not over it yet, you are in the process of recovery and you will have to go through chemo and radio and it will probably make you ill.'

He said he thought I was very practical about it and very brave, and that I was entitled to make the most of my time off. I cried and wondered if Rhodri had sneakily been reading a publication entitled *How to say the right things to your wife with breast cancer*, having gone from one extreme to another himself. I asked him if he thought I was mad, imagining that I was cured. He said that since we saw Mr Monypenny he too felt very positive about it all.

The thing is, I've got another six months of this to face and yet I feel as if it's over, that my story stops here. I just need to focus and remember some of my feelings and think about being calm. I've been given a second chance to look at life anew and I'm bloody well going to take it.

September 27, Wednesday

Rosie was in a chatty mood. She asked me if Rhodri was still up for going to see a counsellor. I said yes, but that I hadn't got round to doing anything about it. Part of the problem is that he's suddenly saying the right things to me and being all sensible. He says I have two good weeks where I am lovely and two bad weeks where I'm not because of my menstrual cycle. When I told Rosie this, she thought it might be interesting to see if he notices a difference with my acupuncture. Arguably Rhodri is the reasonable one and I'm Mrs Irritable. I would, however, have very much appreciated having this conversation with him over the last ten years at some point so that I could have addressed it sooner, is what I said to Rosie.

I told Rosie about my experience with Jane and how I had forgotten about my cancer. I said I wasn't sure if I should say I still have it or I had it. She said she thought that once you've had it, it's something that you always have to think about.

I explained to her that since Mr Monypenny had given me the all-clear I felt demob happy, and I know I have the chemo to come, which is no picnic, but I know it will end and I'm feeling like that's it: I've done cancer, now let's move on.

She told me that I must NOT be blasé about cancer and that things sometimes happen for a reason. This is a warning to me that I have to change things in my life – and she would remind me about that. I do agree with her and she is such a great help, a leveller, a reminder in fact of why I am feeling so positive because I am taking control of my life. I will eat healthily, I will address my relationships and I will never drink copious amounts of alcohol again. I want to feel my senses, I want to be more patient, and most of all I want to be healthy for my children and for ME. So I will endeavour to remember that this is a chance for me to put things right and be thankful for that. Rosie talked about Buddhism and chi and energy, and women being in touch with their inner feelings – and I resolved once again to look it all up on the internet.

September 28, Thursday

Elis is unwell today and is at home with Rhodri. Thank God and Mr Monypenny that I am going to live (fingers and toes crossed) long enough to see my children grow up. Did I say that I would not give Rhodri any instructions on looking after MY children? Let's face it, I carried them and had the 'natural' childbirth, the internal bleeding, stitches and prolapse to prove it. Well, I've changed my mind! My letter may have something in it like, *If your child has a temperature over 100 and has thrown up over the duvet, pillow and his favourite teddy, it might be a good time to take some action.*

I asked Rhodri before I went to bed last night if he had checked on the children. It's a joke between us because before I go to sleep I always check on them to make sure they haven't got temperatures, are not too cold, etc. Paranoid, I know, but I do.

'Yes,' he said. 'I checked on Elis twice tonight,' because Elis has been unwell during the day. 'He's a bit hot but that's because we've had the heating on.' I went upstairs to find Elis had a raging temperature and had thrown up everywhere. In fairness to Rhodri I only saw the sick when

I turned the light on but he was bloody boiling and clearly very unwell. Does our son have to be in a coma before Rhodri does something about it?

I was VERY calm. I moved Elis to a mattress on the floor in our room to keep an eye on him, which also meant neither of us had to sleep directly with him. The last thing I want is for Rhodri to get this bug and give it to me the week before I start chemotherapy. I've waited a bloody lifetime to start already – they will have found a cure for cancer by the time my treatment is done and dusted.

I then quietly chastised Rhodri and gave him some tips on knowing if it is a temperature (the 100 mark on the thermometer) and asked did it occur to him to take Elis's temperature? No, apparently it didn't. 'How can I ever trust you with them?' I said, but not in the usual rasping, snake-like voice, more of a resigned tone. I didn't want to shout in front of Elis (not in front of the children); actually, I didn't want to shout at all. I just thought, Thank God I am here to look after them. I will bring up the subject of children and temperatures at a later date to make sure Rhodri knows what he's supposed to do. I mean, he's been a father for nearly seven years – hello!

I asked Rhodri to sort out the sicky blankets, pillow and duvets as I had done them the day before, when Elis had also been sick, and I want to minimise my contact with Elis's germs as I don't want to get anything before chemo if possible. Anyway we ended up having a screaming row – both of us. Rhodri rarely raises his voice. He's standing there, really pathetic, saying, 'How do I get the sick off?' Now what makes me fucking mad is that in work he is the epitome of cool calm collectedness, in control, making decisions, in short a flexible, intelligent, well-rounded individual. So why, oh why, oh why can't he be like that at home? It's called transferable skills.

I said, 'I don't know. YOU decide how to get the sick off.' I can't even believe I have to have this conversation.

"Scrape it off with a stick, hose the sheet off in the garden or wipe it off. You decide.'

He picks up the bundle of blankets, scattering sick all over the kitchen floor, then proceeds to hose it all down in the garden. Then he comes through the door and everything is soaking wet. 'Don't bring that in like that,' I said, knowing the floor would be awash.

'Well, how on earth am I supposed to get it from the door to the washing machine?' he shouted. I knew the bloody answer – a bucket, a bowl, whatever. I wanted him to work it out for himself, which is what I screamed at him, so he left the stuff at the door and got a bowl.

He gets it all in the bowl and puts it in the washing machine and then starts having a go at me for having a go at him. 'I wasn't shouting at you when you were doing it yesterday,' he said.

'No, that's because I wasn't standing in the door like a pathetic kid saying, "How am I supposed to get it from the back door to the washing machine without dripping". God help you if you are ever stranded on a desert island,' I snarled.

'Well, at least I'm not afraid of spiders,' he said.

I said that was an entirely different argument and he was always pulling the 'pathetic card' when he basically didn't want to do an unpleasant job. If he complained enough, I would give in and do it, and he just didn't like it because for once I hadn't said that I would do it, and that was why he was shouting, because he actually had to do something unpleasant. Do you know what he did when I said that? He smiled, because I had hit the nail on the bloody head – bang to rights.

I sat on the bed with a poorly Elis this afternoon staring at the clouds, and he said, 'Do you know, those clouds will blow all around the world and when it comes to Christmas they come back and snow on us.' I wanted to cry it was so beautiful and sweet. I never ever want him to grow up and be cynical and world-weary or have to worry about anything.

I had my appointment at Velindre Hospital today about my chemotherapy. Rhodri couldn't come with me because he had to look after Elis. I thought it would be fine. It's just a consultation – I could write the book on cancer and chemotherapy; there's really no surprises left for me, I thought.

As I was about to leave, Elis came into the room and said, 'I feel really sick.'

'Oh, poor you,' I said in that way mothers have of saying 'poor you' but not actually meaning it. Suddenly he projectile vomited five times all over the room. On a duvet, on the floor, on the rug, the sofa, the floor again. I pushed him in the direction of the downstairs toilet and he continued to vomit before finally reaching the toilet, at which stage the entire contents of his stomach had already been released so the toilet was no longer much use.

It was a scene of total carnage and I had to leave for the hospital that minute. I looked at Rhodri and we smiled at each other. 'Well,' he said, 'I think I'm about to make amends for my earlier inadequacies, Shell. I'd give anything to be coming to the hospital with you now.'

'I know,' I said, and skipped off merrily, thanking my lucky stars that by the time I returned, the mess would be cleared up.

Velindre hospital is a small place about five minutes' drive from my house – very convenient, although convenience and cancer are not necessarily two words that easily sit together. I arrive and realise it is called Velindre Cancer Hospital. Shit, I'm in a hospital for cancer. I reassuringly note that a woman with no hair in a wheelchair outside the main entrance is smoking a fag.

With every wrong turn and wrong room I entered, trying to find Dr Barrett-Lee's office (as I wasn't really listening to the directions from the receptionist) my tra la la attitude, my 'I've forgotten I have had cancer' attitude was drip-drip-dripping away.

I am confronted by really sick people; I mean people who are clearly dying or who are very seriously ill. These are not people who have shiny hair and manicured nails and a sunny disposition like me. I am talking about wheelchairs and no hair and stretchers. This place should be on the school curriculum as a compulsory trip – not a fag would pass your lips and binge-drinking sessions would diminish. You would want to look after your body and nurture yourself, and thank your lucky stars you are alive, fit and healthy – just as I did, but I have cancer too. This is serious shit. The staff are lovely but almost too lovely; they have seen it all before – the positive, skippy ones like me, the 'they only just manage the stairs' like the woman sitting next to me, the 'we'll give it a go and see if it can help you' and the 'we've done all we can for you'.

I am on the good side of bad, I am on the good side of bad, I am on the good side of bad. I feel people are looking at me because I'm young – well, in this place I am young and bright and cheery and I don't look ill. I look well-dressed and polished and smiling, and I look as if there's nothing wrong with me and I shouldn't be here, and maybe I'm in the wrong place and I should go home and help Rhodri clean the sick up. I won't need to wear gloves in case I catch something off Elis because this has all been a big mistake – sorry about that. But no, my name is called, I am weighed and measured – does chemotherapy shrink you? I am unable at this point to fall in love with Dr Barrett-Lee as his colleague Mr Jacob comes in and examines me. As he prods me about, I wonder whether, if I did have another growth, would it come that quickly? He asked if I was on my own. I told him my son was sick and my husband had to look after him. He methodically went through the treatment. There was nothing that was really new to me but I nodded, not wanting to be rude, while looking at the letter Mr Monypenny had sent to him. I was reading upside down so it was difficult. I said, 'Excuse me, would you mind if I read that letter? It will clear something up for me,' (about the 75 per cent). It said my survival rate with Mr Monypenny's surgical intervention was 75 per cent. I asked Dr Jacob what that meant; he said I was currently at 75 per cent; chemo and radio and Tamoxifen would add on another 14 per cent making a total of 89 per cent.

If they took one hundred women with exactly the same symptoms as me, same age, with negative lymph nodes and tumour removal, adding chemo and radiotherapy and Tamoxifen, then there would be a 90 per cent survival rate over ten years. I told him I thought they were good odds and I would take them. That was the wake-up call I needed. Survival rates and health and being blasé about cancer and not thinking I need to change my lifestyle simply disappeared; by the time he had left the room, the drip-drip-drip of my tra la la attitude to this cancer had finished and I knew I was a cancer patient who was lucky to be alive and I was NOT going to fuck this up for those people who spend their lives looking after people like me – the surgeons, the oncologists, the nurses – as well as for my family, for my husband, for my two beautiful children and for me.

Lizzie is a specialist nurse who works for Cancer Care Cymru, a charity at the hospital which works with cancer patients; when she came in, she explained everything to me again. She gave me a wig prescription which was on Velindre headed paper and said *one wig please* which made me smile. She explained about the cold cap, which is a cap you put on before and after the chemo which can save your hair. I said I would try it but wasn't really that bothered about it. She said if my hair was saved I would have to treat it very gently, that I would have to wash it with baby shampoo and very lightly towel it dry, and that I should only wash it twice, possibly once a week.

'You're joking, I said.

'No', she told me, and said that I could not use a hair dryer.

'You're joking,' I repeated.

'No.'

'What about hair straighteners?'

'No.'

Nor am I allowed to dye it during the treatment, or for six months after.

Oh my God. I've been grey since I was twenty-five, I tell her and without straighteners my hair is curly. So basically I am going to have grey, curly, thin, smelly hair. I'm laughing and saying, 'I'm sorry I'm so vain. I'm sorry there's so many sick people here and all I'm worried about is my bloody hair.'

Lizzie is so kind. She says most women react like me. All I'm thinking is, *one wig please*. I'm thinking Catherine Zeta Jones, *Chicago*, and don't take in another word she says. I hope it wasn't important. I start my treatment on 11 October.

I was humbled by Velindre. Cancer is no great mystery, not really. It is simply a group of cells which decide to work faster than the rest and eventually they will kill you. There is a skill in controlling them and killing them and finding cures against them so that doesn't happen. And these people who work with us, we cancer patients – that is what I am, I am a cancer patient – they are the ones who are the mystery to me. Surrounded by all this illness and suffering and death, they do this work, I suppose, because they see hope in people like me. I feel like a fraud, as if I have less of a cancer than other people, as they are SO ill and I'm not like that – well, not until I'm zapped by the chemo. But I will get better, I have a 90 per cent survival rate in the next ten years, while some of those other people will never leave that hospital. Rosie won't need to remind me about having cancer, for after six months of coming back and forth to this place, I'm not going to forget.

When I got back home, the smelly rug had been hosed down in the garden, washed with disinfectant and was drying in the sun. The duvets had been binned and the floors were clean. Rhodri had indeed, redeemed himself, and I felt so happy to be alive.

October 2, Monday

Elis is off school again. He was fine yesterday so I thought he was OK to go back. However, he was complaining before school that he felt REALLY ill, but I just thought he was trying it on as his sickness had stopped. As a treat, we went to McDonald's after school. I was giving out about McDonald's in the car, saying how crap it was. I said, 'I wouldn't eat it, it is rubbish, but I let you eat it. What sort of mother does that make me?' He replied, 'A great mother.' At midnight I realised he wasn't trying it on, he was really ill, and spent about half an hour throwing up. He was still on a mattress on the floor in our room – the last night just to make sure – so I managed to get him to a bowl before another set of bedding was ruined. He was so ill. Rhodri is in Spain and not back until Thursday. I feel a little bit like I did when I had a new baby. I must have woken about four times in the night and about four times the night before that, to make sure he was OK. Every time he so much as moved I was up checking he wasn't sick – mainly to get to him before he got the bedding. Also, he is usually sick in his sleep, which is very worrying.

The next day, I took him to the doctor – well, nurse practitioner – who checked him very thoroughly and said he has just had a virus, and to keep him off school until he stopped being sick.

God, it's been seven days already. Even he wants to go back to school now. The novelty of staying at home has worn off a long time ago. Although he has escalated up the levels on Lego Star Wars II, so there's an up side to everything.

I am supposed to be going wig shopping with Joanne tomorrow. My mother was on the phone, all mother-like, saying she had got Clive in to look after the farm for the day and I had to go and get that wig and she was going to look after Elis. I said I didn't want to put anyone out, that I had until next Tuesday to get my wig and it would be fine – I would wait until Rhodri was back. 'No,' she said, it was something that had to be done, in the way someone says it when they have to identify a body.

She said, 'You are not putting me out; I am your mother.' God, I hope I'm as self-sacrificing with my children, although hopefully not in the looking-after-the-grandchildren-while-they-go-to-buy-wigs-type way – unless it's for male pattern baldness, then that would be fine. Well, not fine but not life-threatening.

So it was all settled and she is coming down to sit with Elis while Joanne and I go shopping for 'one wig please'. My mother has said she will pay for a more expensive wig. This will be a whole new shopping experience I never thought I would have, but there we go. As she is coming I have tried to tidy up a bit. It's chaotic here and I know what will happen. She'll come down, see the mess and tell my sisters I'm not coping.

I've had a vomiting six year old for a week, have been washing sheets and blankets every day and generally being single mummy while Rhodri is probably having a really hard time (NOT) eating tapas and drinking wine in fab little Spanish bars.

God, I get really resentful when he goes away. I know he works hard and there's not much of a break in the schedule, BUT he's away from home, generally in beautiful locations, generally in another country, and having someone else worry about all his arrangements. He is eating in nice restaurants and most of all sleeping in a hotel room without waking up every hour wondering if his vomiting son has asphyxiated. Try as I might to be the understanding wife, when you are knackered and have two demanding children taking every ounce of your energy, what you wouldn't give for a hard day's filming, a restaurant with tapas, a nice wine and a hotel bed, with clean sheets. Also a bed you could actually get into without having to move the twenty things you put on there earlier thinking stupidly you would put them away later, and without the vomiting six year old on a camp bed on the floor far enough away so you don't catch anything, but not too far so you can't hear him vomiting in his sleep. I suppose I should be grateful because normally when this is happening I am also holding down a full-time job. I'm not sure how I manage that, as the thought of working at the moment is just overwhelming, actually. I'm sure that will change and I will want to go back, but at the moment I can't think about it.

October 6, Friday

My mother came down today to sit with Elis while Joanne and I went wig shopping. I have decided not to have the cold cap because there is a line in the leaflet about hair loss which basically tells you that the cold cap stops chemotherapy going to your scalp, and that in rare cases you can develop cancer of the scalp. Add that to the paranoia I have about every other type of cancer I might get as a result of chemo and radiotherapy, and it's one less thing I can do without.

I don't want to have to go through chemo and still possibly lose my hair and then, every time I have an itchy scalp, think I've got scalp cancer. Also, it's about two and a half hours to have it which is too long to spend in the hospital. I really want to get in and out as quickly as possible.

We went to Howell's department store in Cardiff city centre, where there were some wigs in a window display, so we thought that was it. I told an assistant I had a wig prescription and asked if these were all the wigs they had?

No, she said, they had a specialist wig department, and she directed me to Lingerie. Down a small corridor tucked by the side of the lingerie department in Howell's is the wig department. Unless you had business there, you wouldn't know it existed, it is so discreet. It is a small white room containing various wigs on stands. The woman who works there has obviously seen it, done it, heard it all before and is very professional.

I said I wasn't sure what to go for but was thinking Catherine Zeta Jones in *Chicago*. The woman sat me down and put a bobbed red wig on me, with a fringe almost exactly the same style as mine, in a red colour – my natural colour when I was a child. She adjusted it, gave it a bit of a brush and I was transformed. It was amazing. It was the way I look on a perfect hair day. Joanne started laughing, and said, 'It's perfect – it just looks like your hair.' I couldn't believe it. I took it off and put it back on again to see if I could make it look the same as she had, and I did – it was the same PERFECT HAIR. And that was it: I bought it and came out with perfect hair. All that trauma, all that, 'Oh my God, it's going to look like a wig!' and there it was. You couldn't tell the difference between the wig and my own hair except that the wig was so much better.

Joanne and I then went for a tapas and then we went back to Mum, who couldn't tell the difference between the wig and my real hair, except she said, 'I hate to say it, but it's better than your hair, it's like a perfect version of your own hair.'

'I know,' I said. 'I've finally got the hair I've always wanted and it's a wig. It's amazing.'

Babs came over. She sat down and said, 'Your hair looks

nice,' and I screamed, 'It's a wig!' and she didn't know the difference. She brought a bottle of wine and the children were in bed so we drank it and talked about our cancers. She pulled up her top and showed me her scars and I pulled mine up and showed her mine to illustrate various points we were talking about. We laughed a lot about goodness knows what. She has just had a double mastectomy and I've had an aggressive tumour removed, but maybe that's why we could laugh. Whatever it was about, the wine certainly helped. I love Babs. What would I do without her?

October 7, Saturday

Rhodri came back from Spain this evening and I had my wig on and he didn't notice it was a wig – I'm loving this game! I'd told him on the phone the day before that I'd been to the hairdresser and had it coloured, as the colour is different to what it was before he went away. 'I don't know why I bothered,' I said, setting the scene. 'It's all going to fall out anyway.'

Anyway, after about twenty minutes I said, 'Do you like my hair?' He had raised his eyebrows at it approvingly when he came in, but Elis and Osh took him off into the bedroom to play with them. He said, 'Yeah, it's lovely, really sexy,' and I said, 'It's a wig,' and he said, 'Oh my God,' and I said, 'I know, I want to wear it for ever.' Wigs R Us.

October 9, Monday

Martyn rang earlier. Work seems very stressful, although it never seems like that when I'm there, and I'm more tired being at home than being in work. I'm not phoning people at the moment or having anyone round, I am so tired.

I guess I'm gearing myself up for the chemo mentally and physically. I went to the healthfood shop today to get astragalus – it's in my Suzannah Olivier book. Looked it up on the internet. VERY important in Chinese medicine, as it boosts the immunity, and is very important in chemotherapy, so I have started taking it. Predictably, it costs a fortune. I must check with Rosie that it's OK to take it. I don't want it conflicting with the chi she's working so hard on. The gorgeous man-boy – God of Supplements – in the healthfood shop sold it to me. Ah, he is so lovely, I could definitely do a Demi Moore Ashton whatshisname with him, and he's so nice to my children and he speaks Welsh. I, of course, couldn't have any of his children as I will have withered ovaries or removed ones if the oestrogen-producing time bombs won't die. But like Ashton he could love my children like his own and we could always adopt a Chinese baby or have dogs.

Must do a bit more tidying before my mother comes down casting her aspersions on my ability to cope, little knowing it has nothing to do with cancer. I just can't be bloody bothered, and it's nothing that a husband in the same country, a good night's sleep and two hours to myself wouldn't fix.

October 10, Tuesday

Am I mad? Yes, I am. It's the day before I start chemotherapy and I've got a hangover. I drank almost a bottle of wine last night. Why am I doing this to myself? I wake up feeling like shit with a fuzzy head, then get all irritable. It's my coping strategy, I know, but I am constantly beating myself up about it. I'm supposed to be a picture of health going forward into this when instead I feel as if someone has hit me on the head with a hammer.

I'm trying to hold on to what Alison K said to me the

other day about needing to make sure I have done everything within my control to make sure that cancer doesn't come back. I've forgotten all those thoughts about the sick people in the hospital and about wanting to see my children grow up, all those feelings of desperate hopelessness, thinking I was going to die. I will make an appointment with the counsellor today for next week, as I need someone to talk to, I think.

I'm cashing in on those 'if you ever need anything' offers. Julia is coming Friday so we can go to the Quiz and Curry night at the school – it's one of their fund-raising events. If I'm not well enough, Rhodri will go and I'll stay here with Julia. I just don't want to be left with the children on my own. Kate is coming over Tuesday when Rhodri is at the footie.

This HAS to be a new beginning for me. I think part of my desperation to get started on the chemo is so that it signals a turning point in my life. But only I can do that, it's got to come from me. Not just temporarily because I feel too shit, pumped with toxic chemicals. I have been given a second chance. I can fight this, I can beat this, and I will not let it get the better of me.

I told Elis that the medicine I had to take to make me better, might make my hair fall out and Mummy might have to wear a wig. I don't want to freak him out, so I've mentioned it in passing a few times so he gets used to the idea. He said 'Oh,' fleetingly, then changed the subject immediately to something about Lego Star Wars – his complete obsession. He asked me in the car on the way back from the garage if we could go swimming next week. I said it would be difficult for me to go swimming now as I had to think about my hair falling out.

He said, 'Well, you could sit on the side and watch.' I said I thought it was better if his daddy took him. He said, 'Well, what if he was sat on the side reading a book,' which he wouldn't be, but I didn't interrupt, 'and you had to jump in and save me. Would you be worried about your hair then?'

'No,' I said, 'but that wouldn't happen as Daddy would get a kick up the arse if he took his eyes off you for a minute.'

'But what if he did and he couldn't see me and you were there and you wouldn't jump in in case your hair fell out and you had to wear a wig?'

'Well, Elis,' I said, 'under those circumstances I would then jump in and save you.'

'Good,' he said, 'because your child is more important than your hair and it wouldn't matter then if you wore a wig because you had saved your child.'

'That's right,' I replied, smiling. 'My child is more important than my hair.' I looked in the rear-view mirror and he was nodding sagely. Actually, as I write that I think what a powerful metaphor that is from the mouth of a six year old – if only he knew. Why am I stressing about my bloody hair? I should be bloody grateful I will be alive in ten years to be with my beautiful, clever, happy children.

October 11, Wednesday

Chemo Day number one. It has been eight hours since I had the chemo. We spent over six hours in the hospital today; I had two meals there, seeing various people and waiting around for two hours for the prescription; apparently it will not take as long next time. I was in the canteen and I almost started crying. There was a young boy in there, he was about sixteen, maybe a bit older, I'd seen him having treatment when I was in one of the rooms earlier. I said to Rhodri, 'That little boy is having chemo,' and I started to cry. I said, 'It's OK for me but not for him, it's not fair.' Even if something happens to me, at least I've had forty years of life and given birth to two children, but that young lad had his whole life to live and I pray that he does.

I have not had any side-effects to report so far; I'm still not quite sure what I thought might happen – possibly that I'd keel over on the spot and need an instant blood transfusion and be placed on a life-support machine. The chemo room has about ten people in it and you are sat in chairs. They put a saline drip into you to wash your veins out, then they put another needle into your hand with a tube on and they inject six tubes of the special stuff into your veins; it takes about half an hour.

Chemo is the opposite of childbirth. NO ONE dares tell you what childbirth is actually like, EVERYBODY has a story to tell about chemotherapy and they ALL mainly want to tell you how bad it is.

Ian P in work has a friend who, like me, has two children and had chemo, so I asked him about her. Apparently, she had to have a blood transfusion after her first chemo. Beth, who I met with Babs, can't get out of bed afterwards, and two mothers from the school keep telling me how brave I am, as their fathers have had it. I don't *want* to be brave.

Sandra, who had her op when I had my op, said that after chemo, she felt a bit groggy and was OK the next day, so I'm keeping my fingers crossed I will be like that. Groggy is good, groggy would be excellent. Not being able to move for four days – not so good.

On a positive note, I have had my hair hacked off in readiness for it falling out, for the sum of £11, and it's rather grown on me (no pun intended). I actually quite like it, not that I would wear it in the street as I want people to think my wig is my hair. Rhodri says I look like a cross between Elvis and Sarah my sister. While I keep saying to anyone who will listen that the wig isn't a big deal, the truth is, it *is* a big deal and I should stop pretending otherwise.

Beth was in the hospital on her final chemotherapy treatment. When I saw her she asked me if I am going to go without a wig – she is completely bald and does not wear anything. I said I was thinking about it, just getting used to the idea at the moment, when what I actually meant was, 'No way on God's earth am I going without a wig.' I am completely vain. I think Beth is amazingly honest about the whole thing, plus she has the face to carry it off – petite, not a great big moon-faced owl like me.

Elis looked at my hair earlier and said, 'Is that your hair now?' indicating my new short hair, and I said, 'Yes' and he said, 'Go and put your real hair on,' and I said, 'This is my real hair,' which he wasn't quite sure about. It must be very confusing in his six-year-old head when his mother changes her hair every time she answers the door or pops to the corner shop.

I will wash my wig soon to see if it falls apart. I Googled chemo side-effects and found more or less the same as the hospital says, except not everyone *has* side-effects. I am hoping to be that someone, so watch this space. For now I have the sickness tablets they gave me at the hospital. I also have ginger biscuits and water by my bed and my new book from Amazon, *The Tibetan Book of Living and Dying*. I have only read chapter one, but so far it is very promising, especially the bit that says, *How sad it is that most of us only begin to appreciate our life when we are on the point of death*. Yes, it is sad, and I am going to change all that, I know.

October 12, Thursday

Second day after chemo. Still can't believe I feel relatively normal. I got up and got the children's breakfast and moved some stuff up to the attic and went to lunch with Joanne. I feel a bit nauseous but nothing major. Joanne thought I would be in bed and she would be bringing me soup, and to be honest so did I, but I feel OK. Gill Donovan from Cancer

Care Cymru at Velindre rang me. I really can't fault their service. She has called me twice now; I've told her I am fine and she says if I haven't been sick by now, the chances are I'm not going to be.

I am still taking my anti-sickness tablets and steroids. The nurse who did my chemotherapy at the hospital asked me how I felt about taking steroids and I said I was a bit sceptical but, as they were injecting toxic chemicals into me, steroids were paling into insignificance at the moment so I would take them. I do think they are keeping the nausea under control.

Had a few hours' sleep this afternoon. Gill says Friday is when I might feel a bit flat. Flat is good; not being able to get out of bed would be bad. I have bought Red Bull to stop that flat feeling.

October 13, Friday

Oooh Friday the thirteenth, spooky. Feeling good in myself again today but had a rubbish night's sleep. I think sleeping in the afternoon is not a good idea but I also went to bed at nine so will try to stretch the evening out today. There is a fund-raising Quiz and Curry at the school and I will be going with Rhodri as I feel well enough to attend. I can always leave early.

Julia is looking after the children; she babysat last year when we went and Osh didn't go to bed until 10.30, so I'm hoping it will be better this time, to give her some peace. I am in bed writing this, trying to sleep as I am a bit fuzzy-headed. I'm good otherwise. I am beginning to think that healthy eating (conveniently forgetting my momentary lapses where alcohol is concerned), plus the supplements and acupuncture must be having positive effects on me, as it can't just be a coincidence that I feel so well. I am not stupid enough to think I will escape without some illness, as the little darlings are sure to give me something before the winter is over. I am wearing disposable 'glubs', as Osh calls my gloves, to change his nappies and empty Elis's sick bowls to minimise my contact with their germs, but I will try not to become too paranoid.

Went to my Welsh class, all carrying on as normal. I have to carry a card around with me which says I AM A CHEMOTHERAPY PATIENT on it in big letters: in case of an accident, it tells whoever finds me slumped in a street what to do and what not to do. Mind you, by the time they have gone through my bottomless pit of a handbag past the Tesco and IKEA receipts, lollipops, dummies, dangerous items taken off children for safekeeping, I would have snuffed it. I will endeavour to give my handbag a clear out in order to save my life.

October 14, Saturday

Rhodri took the boys out this morning and I stayed in bed. When they came back I lay there and I heard them all downstairs chattering away, and I thought, That would be them, if I didn't exist any more, if I died. They would be noisy and happy and eating their breakfast and watching television, and although I'd like to think they would miss their mummy, they would survive and they would be happy without me despite that.

As I was thinking this, Osh poked his beautiful head round the door, smiled and said, 'Mummy,' and climbed onto my lap with a Winnie the Pooh book. And I thanked cancer for giving me a second chance in life, for humbling me and for making me realise that life is *not* a rehearsal – and as clichéd as that may be, it is a lesson for us all.

October 16, Monday

Elis wants to be a footballer or a spy when he grows up. I have tried to channel his enthusiasms into a 'proper' job, but if he fails at the first two, he's going to play cricket for England – and who am I to suggest otherwise? I did tell him it is possible to be a spy. I said, 'You could go to college and learn languages and go and live in other countries and be a spy.' He now thinks you go to college, learn Russian, live in Russia and when the Russians aren't looking you sneak up on them – all of which I find very amusing. The Russians won't know what's hit them! Last night, when I was tucking him up in bed, he asked if African people can play football: they are doing 'poor people' in Africa at school at the moment.

Elis says people in Africa should play football because you can earn a lot of money that way. 'You know, football is a very good job, Mum.'

'I know,' I said.

'Well, didn't you ever think about it?'

I assumed he meant as a career option. 'Not, really,' I replied. 'I wasn't that good a football player.'

'But you went to college, didn't you?'

'Yes,' I said

'Well, didn't you ever think to take football?'

So he thinks that you can go to university and be taught how to play like David Beckham, ah, the naivety of youth. I am secretly hoping he will be a builder so he can make a nice little earner thank you very much, like every tradesman that ever darkens these doors. He can do all my DIY in my old age – in my Tenby retirement flat. See? There you go, I do think I might live long enough to retire now, hurrah!

October 18, Wednesday

I had acupuncture with Rosie today. It's been two weeks since our last meeting. She had a week off because she was teaching and then she doesn't do it during the chemo week because the chemo is making enough demands on my body. I had a mini-therapy session with her and said I felt very calm within myself. She said I was different. I explained that I was wearing my new wig (which she thought was my hair – big acupuncture brownie points there), but she said, no, it wasn't the hair, I was simply different. I told her I felt that I was in a different place and that I had changed, and I just wanted to make sure that when I went back to work, this new calm me remained. Also, I told her I was reading *The Tibetan Book of Living and Dying* which she said was a very good book to be reading. I added that Rhodri had said I didn't shout as much, and he too thought I had changed – I AM CHANGED THEN.

So then Rosie did the needles thing. I always forget I actually have to have the needles until she starts doing it. I see it as a little trip to the therapist, then I think, Oh yeah, shit, she's going to stick needles in me. She sticks them in and asks me if I can feel them. I have such a high pain threshold that she really does have to go quite deeply and usually I say in a slightly high-pitched voice. 'Yes, I can feel that!'

I asked her what the needles were hitting and she says they are not actually connecting with bones or sinew but space where the chi is. All very profound, but they certainly connect with something. I told her that I thought the acupuncture was definitely helping and I did feel less paranoid.

I also told her that the last time I came to see her I said I felt I was becoming blasé about having cancer but the trip to Velindre put paid to all that. I was feeling lucky that I was going to come out of that hospital alive and well, and there were many people there who were not as fortunate as me.

Kerry came over with baby Daisy who is sooo cute with little toes in pink sparkly tights – think I will definitely need to have a little dog sometime in the future called Hugo as a baby substitute (hands up who wants a dog – meeee!) I was on the computer after Kerry left, imagining what my invisible dog Hugo would be doing if he were in the room right at that moment. He would lie adoringly at my feet – my loyal companion. I realise I have made Hugo a he – which is interesting as I already have a house of hes and not entirely certain I need another – although this he would be mine, for me and those other hes would have to keep their hands off him – and he would love and adore me, never answer me back or call me a 'stupid cow' as Elis has done on occasion (and as Rhodri probably thinks, but would never dare say) and Hugo would not be singing, 'And it's Cardiff City, Cardiff City FC' from the age of two – although if he did any of those things he would actually be a very valuable dog and would have to appear on *That's Life*, or whatever the equivalent is these days.

Kerry was giving out to Richard C on the phone and I told her I was going to rescue Richard C – although I didn't actually mean it as I would have to look after four men then – as well as my invisible dog. I was feeling very smug because I was so calm and connected to my inner being. Rhodri was very late with Osh and I phoned just to make sure he did actually have him and Osh wasn't in the crèche crying because each one of us thought the other one was picking him up. Rhodri had taken him to his office.

Then Kerry left and by this time it was late and Elis was behaving in a manner that I can only describe as 'little fucker' mode. He was being so naughty and I slapped him on the arse – and then was pissed off with myself for not counting to karma ten.

When Rhodri got back, he said he had been speaking to

someone in work, a woman we both know, and had thought, Oh God, she's going to talk to me about Michelle and it will be a nightmare – but, in fact, he said she was really lovely and understanding, and it was funny that the people who you thought wouldn't be any help, were.

So I said, 'Well, remember she was going through her divorce and I think we connected.' Then he started going on in this really obnoxious manner that that had nothing to do with what he was talking about, saying that he had known her for thirteen years and I didn't know her at all – like any of this mattered one bit – and I just felt so overwhelmingly angry about him speaking to me like that, that I threw my glass of sparkling water over him, right in his face, and walked away. I thought, Fuck where did that come from? He just doesn't listen, he's so fucking wrapped up in what he has to say that what I am trying to say means nothing to him.

Anyway, he was very quiet and I came back and wiped up the water off the floor and didn't say a thing. I was really pissed off that I'd spent the entire day at one with my karma and then in two minutes all the good of the day was undone. He said, 'Sorry,' though as per bloody usual he obviously wasn't sure what he was sorry for.

I then apologised for throwing the water ONLY because I thought it was humiliating for Rhodri, and then he started going on about what I was saying.

I said, 'Look, I'm apologising for throwing the water because it's not a nice thing to do, and it's not good karma, but you were a complete twat so that conversation is not up for further discussion.'

So we ate our food and I decided he could put the footie on. As Elis rightly says, I AM the boss of the house. Overcome with guilt about the sparkling water and the karma thing I apologised again. 'Sorry,' I said, 'about the water.'

'That's OK,' he said. 'It really turns me on when you get

91

like that.'

Ho hum – is there a moral in there somewhere?

October 20, Friday

Me, Osh and Elis are staying with Joanne this weekend as we are having new windows put in and I cannot stand being in the mess or trying to keep Osh from running outside while the men come back and forth. I have left Rhodri to guard the windowless castle while we are away.

October 23, Monday

Had a nice weekend of eating and drinking at Joanne's. Came back this morning and the men were putting finishing touches to the house. The windows look very nice and make the place so much warmer and quieter. So I set to work painting around the sills and the walls around the windows. I started in the downstairs living room and realised the whole thing needed painting so just continued with it.

October 26, Thursday

Finished painting yesterday and it all looks as if it was never any different, but I didn't realise just how tired I was going to be feeling, so haven't really been doing much except sitting in the chair dozing like a pensioner. I need to take it easy as I feel fine but obviously the chemo has an effect. I should try to break the habit of an entire lifetime and conserve my energy, as Helen has advised.

October 27, Friday

After much deliberation I have sent Mr Monypenny a letter. I'm not sure about the appropriateness of sending your surgeon a thank-you card but I feel compelled to do so and I wonder if, because he is a top surgeon and could be seen as a bit scary, many people do thank him. So here it is:

> *Dear Mr Monypenny,*
>
> *I wanted to write to you personally to thank you for everything you and your team have done for me over the past few months. Obviously, having saved my life, there is a gratitude that words cannot express and you have put me well and truly on the road to recovery because of your brilliance as a surgeon.*
>
> *A diagnosis of cancer is devastating for anyone and their families but I don't really view it in those terms, as it has given me a chance to re-evaluate my life in a way that I may never have had the opportunity to do otherwise. You and your team are instrumental in buying me the time when I can put all these new thoughts into practice and live life with my husband and two young children with renewed vigour because of this experience.*
>
> *Throughout my treatment you made me feel as if I mattered, as if I was unique, and you listened to what I had to say and respected it. In short, you made me feel like I was an individual, not just another patient in a very large case-load. It is also those qualities that make you a brilliant surgeon.*
>
> *Thank you.*

I bought a very nice John Knapp Fisher card and sent it immediately in case I changed my mind.

October 30, Monday

Ah, shit, bugger, shit, my hair is coming out in handfuls almost three weeks to the day since I had my first chemo and there was I, thinking I was fucking invincible. At this rate it will all be out by the end of the week. I don't like it, I want it back. I am going to look like shit shit shit. Rhodri said, 'Just think how great Kylie looks, now her hair has grown back.' I did point out that I was about six dress sizes bigger than Kylie and that she is probably one of the few women on the planet who can pull that off and she is a pocket-sized princess of pop superstardom. The only other one is Sinead O'Connor and she had a bit of a breakdown. And all those women out there who go about without wigs or scarves, I admire them deeply but I REALLY WANT MY HAIR BACK.

October 31, Tuesday

Trick or treat. Went to hospital this morning to get my bloods done, so don't have to wait the six hours I waited last time. I just go in at 11 a.m. tomorrow and they do the chemo straight away. So I went at 8.30, got the bloods done and then walked into Whitchurch to get the car taxed and stock up on trick-or-treat goodies, which I had forgotten about. I was in the post office when the hospital rang. They said, 'It's the hospital here.' I thought, Which hospital? What's wrong? Forgetting I myself was under the doctor at a hospital. They said, 'You are supposed to see the doctor and a student is waiting for you.'

'Oh,' I said, 'I didn't realise that.' So I walked back with all my trick-or-treat goodies and my pumpkin.

I saw Gill Donovan, who smiled. I'm sure she's seen it all before. Her manner is a bit like Rosie's – all calm and reassuring and she makes you feel grown-up and that what you say matters. She said the bloods were fine and I was very quick leaving. I thought, Let's get out of here as quick as you like. I didn't want to be around all those sick people. In my mind I have distanced myself from them, not really identifying myself as one of 'those sick people'. I am still very tired at the moment; I think painting the new windowsills was a bit over-ambitious. Also, I went out with Alison K and Neil on Saturday and had a drink and, although it wasn't excessive, I'm not used to it any more. I never thought I would be saying that, but there it is. So in a way I'm glad the next session is tomorrow, as I will take it easy for a week now.

The children are in school and crèche, so I need to slow down and stop thinking I can do everything in a week. I've got months to do gardening and clean out those cupboards and do the front lawn, but in my head I'm trying to get everything done in a week. So SLOW DOWN is the motto.

I have agreed to have a third-year student called Rachel follow me through chemo. They want the students to follow someone who has been diagnosed with cancer, to let them get a feel for the emotional and practical side of dealing with it, as well as the medical side.

God, she was so young and next year she will be let loose on real people. She asked me when I was diagnosed with cancer and I thought, Shit, I hate that word, for all the bravado of saying to Rhodri that I don't know why people don't talk about cancer because a lot of them are going to get it in their lifetime. The truth is, people rarely mention the word when they ask you how you are, and I guess I rarely use it either. I say 'when I was diagnosed' or 'my illness' so it is a stark reminder when someone actually reminds you that you have cancer.

I was talking to her about not really having the opportunity to dwell on it that much, because the children take up most of my time, but the truth is that in your twenties you haven't got a clue about life and responsibilities and children, and still probably think you will live for ever, despite seeing death on a regular basis.

You basically need to live a bit and have trials and tribulations to have a deep understanding about what people go through.

Joanne and my mother (Kim and Aggie as I call them) came to clean the house today. They insist it will be their regular thing the day before I go in for treatment, so the house is immaculate and I am sitting here with a glass of wine, because I know Rhodri would look at me with his disapproving stare if I had one tonight. I feel very warm-cheeked and might have to go and have a lie-down in a minute. I really could do with a little sleep.

Sarah had a biopsy for a lump in her breast. There is a higher chance of you getting breast cancer if a sister has had it. They didn't want to tell me, but anyway, she had a biopsy and it was all OK. Joanne has also got checked out and Julia is going soon. I thank God I haven't got daughters. I know men can get breast cancer and that's usually passed on through the maternal line, but it is rare.

Went to the zoo yesterday with the boys and Rhodri, and Neil and Jay and Erin, and had a really lovely day. Life should be like that all the time – quality time with friends and family. Osh and Elis were drawing pictures and I went for a sit-down in the front room and Osh decided to do a Picasso in red pen all over my newly painted walls – that'll teach me to be so house-proud. He was hysterical when Rhodri told him off, because no one ever tells him off, and he was sobbing, 'I want my mummy, I want my mummy.'

I asked him this morning who did it and he said it was Elis, then proceeded to spit on it and try to rub it off with his sleeve, but it will take more than a bit of spit to get that off. I will have to get the paintbrushes out again.

Osh went off to crèche this morning dressed as a pumpkin and Elis went to Kid's Club in his new tracksuit, not wanting to wear his Halloween T-shirt. I think he thought it was a little beneath him, but he wants to be a vampire later. I have just carved out my pumpkin, but as there were only very small ones left in the shop, the big ones having been bought by the good mothers who remembered earlier, the nose and mouth have sort of melded into one. I figure that Elis and Osh will be so high on toffee apples and Haribos it will take them about two days to come down, and a nose and mouth sort of melding together on their pumpkin will be the last thing on their sugar-crazed minds.

My hair continues to come out and now I'm facing the fact I will be an 'egg-head' as Elis calls people with no hair. This wig is quite tight, I think that is what makes it so good. Gill in the hospital said she wasn't sure that it was a wig, she had to have a really good look, and she sees people with wigs all the time. Although maybe she says that to all the egg-heads who pass her way.

It's just quite shocking when it comes out, no matter how much you prepare yourself for it. Think I will put a scarf on as the wig gives me a headache after a while – or maybe that's the glass of wine!

November 1, Wednesday

Second chemo today. I'm an old hand at this now. My hair is still falling out. Rhodri says I look very attractive in my scarves, like a Russian peasant; he is a big fan of *Dr Zhivago*. Because it was Halloween last night, Elis thought I was dressed as something. I had a black dress on and a bright pink headscarf. I told him I was a Russian witch – he'll think I'm in permanent costume.

Helen called last night, I haven't heard from her for a bit and she said my hair will start growing back between the fourth and fifth sessions. I told her I didn't like to ask them about it at Velindre because it's so trivial.

Had a nice Halloween night with ducking apples and ducking chocolate (my invention) and generally they ate enough crap to fuel one of those sugar-powered cars – if in fact sugar-powered cars exist and I haven't just made that up. I have realised that I focus very much on negative incidences in my life. For example, we had a really lovely evening, then Elis was very tired and didn't want to go to bed which was fine as it's half-term and he can go whatever time he likes – which usually means falling asleep on the sofa at nine o'clock. Anyway, he sneezed on me and that's a real trigger for me as he's full of cold and I am of course slightly paranoid about picking colds up, so I told him off and said it was a rude and disgusting habit. He then called me a silly cow. I said, 'Don't call me a stupid cow, that is hurtful.' He said, 'I didn't call you a stupid cow, I called you a silly cow,' and it sort of went downhill a bit for five minutes. Dr Tania Bryer's toes would be curling reading this. I know I should have walked away. Then Kate rang and asked if I'd had a nice evening and instead of saying yes, it was lovely, which it was for the three hours of ducking apples and ducking chocolate and watching a film, I focused on the five minutes in which I had a row with Elis. Why is that? There must be a psychological explanation. And the more I thought about it, the more I realised I actually do that quite a lot. I fool myself into believing I am a glass half-full when the reality is, I am a glass half-empty.

I must ring the counsellor; I'm sure I can be helped by her. That's not a good trait to have and I think it's like that with the cancer; I am outwardly positive but inwardly perhaps somewhere I do think I'm still going to die. I am trying to accept the inevitability of death (à la Tibetan style) as that is a good spiritual place to be. I really need to spend more time reading *The Tibetan Book of Living and Dying* – will do so now.

I feel much less tired today, which is good. Helen said that although I might feel well and might want to catch up on all those jobs, I must not forget that I was having treatment which was killing my white cells and would make me very tired. I have a long way to go and I really must take it easy, she told me, so I will listen to her as she is a nurse and sometimes they do know best.

I've just been interrupted by the 'tree man' who has come to give me a quote on pruning our trees. They haven't been done for two years and I feel a responsibility to keep them in shape. I used to think they did this themselves, but apparently this is not the case and they need regular pruning, care and attention. I had not realised this when I took on a garden that has eight trees and a very hefty hawthorn bush in it.

The tree man is so young he still has spots. I thought he must be the apprentice and tried to elicit gardening knowledge from him, which wasn't exactly flowing. I eventually just asked him outright if he knew what he was doing and he said he'd been doing it since he was seven with his dad and he's just started up on his own. He had a sweatshirt with his company name on and his company details on his van, so he looked the part if nothing else. Plus he had tree bark on his trousers so he must be doing something to someone else's trees too.

The last people who came to give me a quote never bothered to ring me back, and I'm not getting on a ladder up in those trees, some of which are as big as this house, plus that hawthorn bush nearly hospitalised me with the scratches the last time I did anything to it, I thought I'd give him a go – he's got to start somewhere. I figure that, like a bad haircut, if he massacres them they'll grow back and for £180 it's worth the risk. He has assured me he is insured

November 3, Friday

Aargh! Once again for effect – aargh! I need an anger management course or counseling. All I have to do is pick the phone up, I've got the bloody woman's name and number. I don't know what's wrong with me – oh yes, I've got cancer – oh no, that's a poor and shoddy excuse maybe I'm menopausal – that is one of the side effects of chemo. If women are near to menopause age, although I read that's about fifty-something, you could begin the menopause on my treatment. BUT that is a poor and shoddy excuse for clouting my son. Elis has been a bit of a git these last few days. Maybe my illness is affecting him.

When Rhodri went to Elis's parents' evening (five minutes per child), Miss Smith said Elis was great at reading and maths but wondered if things at home were affecting him as sometimes he refused to do as he was told. Rhodri said he thought not. I said to Elis it was OK to say no, but he should give Miss Smith a reason why he didn't want to do something.

My mother was shocked by this and says he shouldn't question authority. I thought yes, and that attitude means that I am now frightened of my own shadow. I said I was glad he questioned authority.

However, I clearly didn't mean my own authority when I said this, as my word is law, and when he is disobedient I just get annoyed and smack him. He hates homework. He says and this is the first real bit of homework he's ever had to do. Thank God I'm learning Welsh because if you couldn't read Welsh you wouldn't stand a chance. Really I don't know how parents manage who can't speak Welsh or who aren't learning, unless they've got really bright children.

He refused to do it; he was being silly. The homework asked what he had done the previous week and he said he wanted to write and draw about going to the toilet on his holidays. Then he had a screaming tantrum over me turning the Playstation off, which Rhodri had just let him go on. I said to Rhodri at 8.30 this morning, 'Give him breakfast, make him do his homework, then his piano practice, then Playstation.'

This is what he actually did: piano practice, no breakfast, as he thought I said I had given it to him, then he let Elis play on the Playstation and could not understand why Elis refused to do his homework. So then he left me with a surly, hysterical child and went to work – FUCK HIM.

It's Rhodri I'm angry with and I've taken it out on a six-year-old boy. Next time I will count to bloody ten or give myself a slapping.

Anyway, Elis has gone off to play football for the day with Jay, so maybe that will get rid of some of his manic energy, and when he comes back, we'll calmly draw him going to the toilet on his holidays. I'm taking him up to the farm to stay for two nights with my parents. In fairness, he's seen very little of us this week, what with Kids' Club, footie, and now my parents, apart from when we went to the zoo last week. But I didn't know how I was going to be after my second chemo, so I needed to err on the side of caution and take it easy. I still feel a bit of a fraud, as I am very well, if a bit tired.

November 4, Saturday

I had a varied night's sleep once again. I had a nightmare and was doing one of those silent dream screams where you know you are screaming but nothing is coming out – it was quite harrowing.

I mentioned to my sister Julia that I was glad of a break from Elis as he had been very trying over the last few days. She and her husband both work in child protection. I said I sat there the other day thinking I can really see how people can hit their children and the next thing I knew I'd done it. I said I only tapped him, but it was a knee-jerk reaction.

They had just returned from a week in Spain with Lloyd and she said on the fourth day she went to bed crying because Lloyd was so naughty and she couldn't do anything with him. Apparently, Martin had tapped him too one night at dinner and she said, 'Don't start doing that or we might not know when to stop.'

Hurrah! Even professional workers in the field have children who drive them to distraction. It is the school holidays – I guess it is par for the course to be a little bastard for your parents. Thinking about it, I can remember being really naughty with my aunt and uncle who used to look after me (I hope Elis never reads this). Had a long conversation with Kate about life and the universe, mainly about naughty children and going off the rails, and how we had to wait for bloody everything, and how we strived to achieve things because we didn't have them, and were we doing our children a disservice by giving in to their every bloody whim? Probably. We were like two middle-aged women, which I guess we are. Dad has come to collect Osh for the night – Elis is already at the farm – so it's just me and Rhodri . . .

November 5, Sunday

Has the world gone mad? My dear husband appears to be normal. Had a normal day with my normal husband, and went for a pizza and had normal conversations, then came home and watched telly, sitting together like normal people. We went on a beautiful walk somewhere we've never been before. We usually go walking around a lake in Penarth, but we saw a track and took it. It was open fields and woods, a beautiful, cold, crisp day and it was lovely. He asked me how Kate was and I was relaying our conversation about children today having it all, saying I was talking about my teenage niece Emily and my step-nephews Rhys and James and teenagers (or Ninjas as Elis refers to anyone you call a teenager – he thinks teenagers are Ninjas because of Teenage Mutant Ninja Turtles) in general and their lot in life today.

Rhodri was coming out with all these pearls of wisdom about children and parenting and how yes, they did have everything given to them, but their freedom had been taken away from them. We both had childhoods where we spent hours and hours away from our parents, in rivers and up mountains and running across fields, a freedom our children could never have in a city – that's the price to pay for living here.

Then we went for a coffee in the Washington Gallery and had lovely cake and had more normal conversations about Welsh art, then we went to the Cancer Research shop and bought some really great books for Elis, *Life on Earth* and a fantastic 1950s children's illustrated encyclopaedia. Rhodri said it was for me, not Elis, as I liked it so much. Then we went home and had a little lie-down and read the papers and it was all really pleasant.

Later we went to Llandaff village, to the Italian restaurant, and again we talked about lots of different things; it was all really nice.

I guess taking yourself away from the children and rediscovering what it is you liked about your partner in the first place is a reality check we could have more often. I said on the way back from the restaurant (between rocket-fire from various bonfire parties) that people usually find something in their partners that's missing in themselves. You know, they want to fill in the gaps. I said, 'You spoke Welsh and were musical, and had been to a good college, and had a nice house and actually talked about wanting children, and all those things appealed.' I also thought that he was very handsome, of course. He considered his reply –

for a bit too long, I thought – and said, 'You're just incredibly sexy and beautiful and very intelligent; that's what I saw in you. Now come on, let's go. I'm desperate for a pee.' Ho hum, it looks like we love each other very much.

November 6, Monday

Rhodri has been working in St David's for a few days. My lovely mother had plans in place for when Rhodri is working away, which I was very grateful for at the time as I didn't know how the chemo would affect me but, apart from the first three days, I have been able to look after the children by myself. In reality, that's getting them up at eight (they won't wake before that, unless it's the weekend of course when you want a lie-in, and then they are up at seven), dispatching them to school and nursery by nine and then picking them up, which I can do at six, but it's usually about four thirty and they are both in bed by eight – so it's not exactly stressful, although Osh took it upon himself to have his first tantrum last night.

I don't think he was himself though, although I know this is a middle-class parents' excuse for a child's bad behaviour. I had cooked a fabulous lamb dinner and made gravy (Rhodri does not allow me to make gravy – I am beginning to question his authority on this) and wanted Osh and Elis and me to sit down and chat and eat our dinner together. As per bloody usual, nothing worked out as planned. I turned the telly off in the front room and said Osh could watch telly while he had his dinner in the kitchen. He absolutely refused to come; he wouldn't move and wanted to have his food in front of the telly in the living room, a habit that it took two years to get Elis out of.

We were so desperate for him to eat that we would have stood on our heads naked as long as Elis ate something. Of course, I know now that it was our parenting rather than his eating that was the problem. So the upshot of that is we have endeavoured with Osh to get him to eat at the table, NEVER make a fuss if he doesn't want something and NEVER spend half an hour discussing eating and cajoling him into doing so. It doesn't work. The best cure is chill out. They will eat eventually – oh, and don't give in and give them any old crap, that doesn't work in the long term either. Tonight, Elis didn't like the gravy. He said it four times; after the fourth time I said, 'I know you don't like the fucking gravy, stop saying that.'

When he grows up a foul-mouthed, hoodie-wearing yob, and I wonder where it all went wrong, I must remember this. I must stop swearing in front of him, well, actually *at* him – is it child abuse? The theory is that if they hear their parents swearing, they will think it's so uncool that they won't do it themselves. Even I am not convinced by this argument. (I must smile at a hoodie next time I see one – it is clearly not his fault). So Elis and I ate our dinner in the kitchen while Osh screamed hysterically in the front room, which was not, of course in the least bit stressful for me, oh no.

When dinner was finished I went in the living room, put the telly on (basically Dr Tania would be turning in her House of Tiny Tearaways), sat there and cajoled Osh into eating his dinner – which he did, in fairness, and enjoyed it without complaining about the fucking gravy, probably because he can't really articulate this yet. But basically it all happened on his terms, watching his programme, eating on the sofa – whatever.

Elis was rude to his music teacher, Miss Fran – who is a really lovely woman. She comes to the house every Tuesday and she says he is very musical, which I don't doubt for a minute, as he has a perfectly beautiful singing voice. He was really naughty and in the end I went in and intervened. She said she doesn't like to shout at them – she's just started on her own as a teacher. My God, she's got a lot to learn if she's teaching six year olds piano.

'He needs a firm hand,' I said. 'Please feel at liberty to tell him off.' Jesus Christ, music teachers scared the shit out of us in our day, you wouldn't dare be rude to them.

She said he was in a funny mood and didn't listen. I heard him deliberately playing off-key. I know nothing about music and yet I know he was taking the piss because before she came he was playing and it was perfect. She said, 'You often find very musical children behave like that,' making out he was this creative genius. No, he's just a little sod, I wanted to say.

We never push him really, but I am beginning to think he does have a talent and so I want to persevere. A lot of Rhodri's family are musical. Rhodri has a music degree and is obsessed with music. Sioned, Rhodri's aunt, is a concert harpist and a wonderful piano player, and Rhodri's mother is a very accomplished pianist, so I do think it's in his genes.

As a child my grandmother had a piano in her front room and I would spend hours playing it, learning by ear very complicated pieces. I cannot for the life of me understand why someone didn't give me piano lessons.

Even if Elis isn't the most accomplished pianist on the planet, if he has a grounding in music it will be with him for ever. If nothing else, he'll always be able to play 'Happy Birthday' on the piano! He is Miss Fran's youngest student and is better than children two years older than him. I think I'll sit in the room next time, just to make sure my creative genius listens.

November 7, Tuesday

Part of me wishes I would wake up one day and be bald. Tibetan monks don't have hair, do they? No, I don't think they do, and somewhere in the back of my mind a little cog is turning that says that's to do with avoiding vanity – get rid of your hair and you never have to worry about it.

Except real life's not like that. For instance, Gail Porter loses her hair and it's all over the papers, so even though she doesn't have a bad hair day, she does have a bad hair day, get it? Profound. Anyway, if I am bald or 'bold' as Elis calls it, then that's it – start again. At the moment though, I've basically got a head full of dead hair; touch it and it falls out, brush it and it falls out but not quite enough to think, Fuck it, and shave it off in some momentous gesture.

I have my dark brown hair, which is peppered with grey, flat to my head where my wig has flattened it and I dare not touch it as it falls out. I have even begun to forget about washing it. Yesterday I could smell something funny all day and kept thinking, 'What's that smell?' then realised it was my hair. I can't remember the last time I washed it.

Anyway, I washed it this morning in the shower and half-hoped that with one touch it would all come out and that would be it. When chemo is over then I would start again with a glorious head of hair looking like I had just stepped out of a salon, because I would be lucky to have the chance to start again rather than patching it up continually (a bit like my front lawn).

I'm so very very excited about Christmas that I went to the Cancer Research shop and spent £15 on cards. I thought about not sending real cards and sending ecards instead, but relented. On the back of the cards it says, *Together we'll beat cancer*. Yes, thank you, Cancer Research, we WILL beat it.

I am giving £12 a month to Cancer Research. I give £8 to Greenpeace and was thinking about stopping that and giving it to Cancer Research, but do worry about the Amazon rainforest a lot so I'm in a bit of a dilemma.

I will be writing out Christmas cards and wrapping presents over the next week. I'm so bloody organized. Then I can concentrate on the colour scheme for my Christmas table (am thinking burgundy). I have a beautiful cinnamon and clove Christmas candle from Marks & Sparks which I will light tonight.

I feel slightly liberated as it is getting close enough to Christmas to dare speak about it. I'm thinking of getting my parents Sky Plus as my father goes on ad infinitum about not giving money to Rupert Murdoch, so this way he gets the telly he wants, can record programmes for my mother, doesn't have to pay Murdoch and we get something decent to watch when we are up there.

Elis thinks it's a most marvellous idea as we could have the family package for them, which has all the children's channels. I've bought Elis and Osh Marks & Spencer's slightly sanitized version of the nativity which plays 'Away in a Manger' (or Away in a Manager as Elis read it); you sing along to it. I know Rhodri will be scathing about it and that's partly why I bought it, as Elis needs no excuse to be in the God squad with me. I just think, as I have said to Rhodri, Christian values are sound values to have in life and he can't argue with that.

I've been reading it to Elis and Osh in bed every night before Rhodri comes back and it's their favourite book, especially as at the end you press a button and it plays 'Away in a Manger' and you sing three verses. Elis is particularly taken with this and even wants to learn it on the piano for Miss Fran!

We lay in bed last night and Elis, in his perfectly beautiful singing voice, sang, 'The cattle are lowing, the baby awakes, but little Lord Jesus, no crying he makes. I love Thee, Lord Jesus, look down from Sky Plus, and stay by my side, until morning is nigh.'

We laughed so hard, the pair of us, our sides ached and tears were in our eyes.

November 8, Wednesday

I keep singing to the children that Eartha Kitt song, 'Santa baby, put a present under the tree for me . . . ' It's stuck in my mind now and I'm singing it over and over again. The only thing is, in my mind I sing 'Cancer baby, put a present under the tree for me' which is a bit disconcerting. Actually, a 100 per cent cure would be just the thing, please. Thanks. Failing that, I'll have a digital camera.

November 10, Friday

Chemotherapy has a smell to it. The first time I had chemotherapy I thought that I would have to throw away my red duvet cover with all the pretty white flowers on it because of the smell. I kept asking Rhodri if he could smell something but he couldn't. I suppose the smell comes through your skin, does it? I don't know, maybe it's like garlic; all I know is that about four days after chemo I have to change all my bedding because I think it has a smell to it. By five days the chemo is more or less out of your system, I think. Should I know all these things?

I did ask Gill about that because you can pass the chemo on through your bodily fluids; so it can kill the fast-dividing cells of other people in extreme circumstances. I have visions of Osh's cells (no one else's for some reason) being zapped and the poor wee mite fading away before my eyes like a balloon from which the air has been let out.

One of the pieces of advice they give you in the chemotherapy booklet from Velindre is to flush the toilet – something I tend not to do if I wee (save the planet etc – don't flush unless you are forced, as my mother says). Now I am flushing left, right and centre and washing away the planet.

What chemotherapy smells like is death. My mother and

her sister Janet nursed my Auntie Beatie, who had lung cancer, until she died. So I know what death smells like. Since Auntie Beatie died I have been unable to have any air fresheners in the house as they remind me of her dying.

Trying to mask the smell of death is impossible and also rather pointless. It's not faeces or sick or body odour; it is a smell of death. When I go into my bedroom in the mornings after I have had chemotherapy, I feel the need to open the windows and change the bedding to rid my room of the smell.

The way I reconcile it is that it is killing the cancerous cells – that is where the death smell comes from. It is short term and won't last for ever, and I am dying, we all are; this will just help me live a little bit longer so my two children will have their mummy until they are old enough to cross Zebra crossings, boil eggs and iron clothes, then they can go out into the world as fully developed individuals with my duvet of love wrapped around them.

November 11, Saturday

Alison W, my neighbour, had her baby on Thursday – another little girl, a sister for Erin. I have two Alisons and Erins in my life, which is fine when they are apart, confusing when they are together, and even more confusing when I am talking to Rhodri about either Alison or Erin. So I refer to them in conversation as Alison K and Alison W. Alison W's Erin goes to crèche with Osh and her husband works at the BBC. Before we moved here I would dream of having neighbours with babies who I could talk to and go for walks with, with our pushchairs. When we lived in Canton we were the only people in the street who had a baby. People either had grown-up children or they were elderly, and no one was really that friendly, so I felt a bit isolated. The way you meet women with babies is to move to housing estates and you have instant friends, people in the same position as you, but we didn't want to move outside of Cardiff. We also wanted an old house, so when we moved here and I saw our neighbour had a baby the same age as ours, it was like a dream come true. We have been really good friends ever since. The upshot of all this is that Alison W having her baby means I got to do my favourite bit of shopping – baby girl shopping. Having had two boys and having had all Osian's clothes passed to me from my two sisters and Kerry, I never have to buy him any clothes at all, ever, not a thing. He is the cheapest baby in Cardiff, I tell Rhodri. Some of the clothes he has were originally Elis's, which have been around four other children and are now coming back to Osh. I wholeheartedly subscribe to recycling clothes. I was going to give Alison W all Osh's clothes if she had a boy so now they've reached the end of the line – although I think my mother's friend's daughter has a child a bit younger than Osh, so I can pass them on there.

I bought the new baby a pink tutu skirt, shamelessly girly, with a pink bow on the front and sequins, a white cardigan embroidered with roses, and pink tights. I want to wear the cardigan myself, it is so beautiful – I hope Alison W likes it. What with Alison W's baby (no name yet) and baby Daisy, I can satisfy my pink baby purchasing for many birthdays to come.

I don't feel sad about not being able to have another baby. There was a time when I obsessed about it after Osh. Obviously, having my own baby isn't possible now on two counts. Firstly, I physically might not be able to have one and I know, having an oestrogen-receptive tumour, that pregnancy would not be good, but I am not certain about that as women do have children after they have had cancer. But I think for me, personally, I wouldn't want to bring any child into my family thinking I might have to go through all this again. I need to gather my strength to look after my two

111

boys and myself should I have to face it again in the future. Please God though, let that not be the case.

I met Kate yesterday to go shopping and she was telling me about someone she works with who has had breast cancer twice. She's just got it again, but they had told her it would come back within ten years – although it has only been four years.

I didn't know they could say that and wonder what sort of cancer it is. She didn't have chemo the first time but is having it the second time.

How do they know it's going to come back? How can they tell that? I'm going to ask Gill about that just to put my mind at rest. I found myself thinking yesterday that maybe all my family know something about my treatment and know I'm going to die, that's why everyone is being so kind to me, and then I checked myself for being so ridiculous. They can't do that these days, can they? Unless you are about ninety or something?

I wondered how Kate's friend could live every day of her life for the last four years not thinking, Today the cancer will come back, since a medical professional had told her that it would.

The only way I can reconcile living with the paranoia is knowing that the odds for this tumour are in my favour and, if I get another one, I'm already in the system; I am being checked, they will get that early too and those cancerous cells floating round my body will be zapped. However, it will always be a little niggle at the back of my mind.

Anyway Kate and I were in Borders for about two hours and we both independently wound up in the self-help section and bought the same book: *Ten-Minute Life Coach*. I had it in my hand and turned around and there she was with it too. We instantly recognised ourselves in the parts we read. *Good people are the most likely to dislike themselves. The reason for this is that they desire to do good. They feel compelled to be good, to do the right thing, to cause no harm or suffering to another living being. This might sound a little pious, but that's how it is and I suspect you may be recognizing yourself here,* at this point we are both nodding vigorously, *and the reason they are most likely to dislike themselves is simply this – good people are always the most sensitive, thin skinned and open to suggestion. This is acutely the case when they are children and at their most vulnerable. Their tendency to blame themselves for anything and everything that goes wrong in their world and the world at large takes root*.*

We both said in unison: 'I'm buying this.'

I have great hope for the life coach, PLUS I forgot that my friend Mari with whom I had lunch the other day sent me an information pack on becoming a life coach. I feel a new career coming on here – will check out Mari's pack right now.

*Ten-Minute Life Coach, by Fiona Harrold Copyright © 2002 Fiona Harrold

November 12, Sunday

Me and Kerry and baby Daisy went to see Alison W's new baby, who didn't have a name when we arrived but Alison and her husband Mark had called her Angharad by the time we left. She is tiny and quiet. Kerry and Alison and I talked about the older siblings being a complete nightmare when they were babies, not sleeping, feeding constantly and generally taking the piss out of us. Elis slept in our bed for nearly five years, so when Osh came along I bought the queen of sleeping babies' book – *The New Contented Little Baby Book* by Gina Ford – and from two weeks old I followed it to the letter.

The result is a child who sleeps independently, in fact doesn't like being in bed with us at all and sleeps for thirteen hours a night. Apart from a few odd nights when he was teething he has been perfect. He doesn't cry, have tantrums, always goes to sleep perfectly, no problems with food and doesn't need the twenty-four seven attention that his brother demands.

Alison W looked very well, and although baby Daisy and baby Angharad are sweet, I would be too tired to have another.

November 13, Monday

I have shaved off all my hair. It was not a traumatic, life-changing moment – it's just me without hair. I look like Paul with whom Rhodri works; he's handsome and has his head shaved. My hair has been dead for weeks and if I run my fingers through it, most of it comes out. There are some patches that don't, but I figured what's the point of keeping those, because when it grows back it will be grey and dark brown in places and then I will want to colour it so it will be three different colours and different lengths. So I shaved it all off. I asked Rhodri if he thought I should get rid of it and he said if it was him, he would. Plus I'm fed up of hoovering hair up all of the time. Elis was on his Playstation, Rhodri was in London and Osh was hiding in the washing basket in my bedroom and is two and away with the fairies, so I don't think he will be too traumatised by it and have to have counselling when he is older.

I knew Elis would be a petrified zombie for at least an hour on his Playstation until I told him he needed a break, otherwise he would have a fit seeing me do it. As it turned out, he didn't move from the Playstation and has not noticed any difference because if I'm not wearing my wig I am wearing a turban which is a black, tight-fitting hat, so he never sees me without either of those. Osh watched with great interest from the washing basket as I did it. I got the hair clippers that I use to butcher Osian and Elis's hair and

114

just shaved it all off and Osh kept looking at me and saying periodically, 'Mummy's hair's gone. Mummy's hair's gone! *Mummy's hair's gone*!' Each sentence with a different intonation, going slightly higher each time.

November 14, Tuesday

Have eaten a whole box of Black Magic to myself. I don't even like Black Magic. Gwyneth and David over the road gave them to me. I have the keys to their house in case their alarm goes off when they are away for a few days, and they gave me the chocolates 'for the children'. Within two minutes of having them in the house I had opened them and eaten an entire layer – even the coffee one.

Am picking Elis up from school today to do reading and piano in a calm environment after last week's fiasco when he was rude to Miss Fran; I want to avoid a repetition of that at all costs.

I have promised Elis an electric guitar for his eighth birthday if he practises the piano and is not rude to Miss Fran and listens to her for the next year. He has always wanted an electric guitar so this is a good bribe, plus secretly I'm hoping he will become a pop star and keep me in the lifestyle to which I feel I deserve to be accustomed. He is handsome and has a beautiful singing voice and is very musical. I am of course a bit biased but surely these are the foundations for becoming a pop star? I will definitely encourage him in this career path as having two degrees has never done me any bloody good or made me any money. He can buy me a bungalow in West Wales overlooking the sea and I will definitely have a real dog not an invisible one called Hugo, and sod what Rhodri says about dogs; he'll just have to take an antihistamine tablet every day.

Kate is coming over tonight with her friend Cathy, the

woman who has had breast cancer twice. Kate has been talking to her about me and Cathy wants to chat to me about chemo and wigs, since she didn't have chemo first time round. I've been thinking that the main thing about cancer is to try and turn it around into something positive, which I think I am doing. Once you have it there's no point bemoaning the fact. There's nothing you can do about it, so you have to use it as a positive force for change. I will omit to tell Cathy that I can still sink a bottle of red in one sitting.

Rhodri came back late last night and when I woke up this morning, I said, 'I've shaved my hair off,' and showed him. I said, 'I look like Paul.' He just smiled and had to zip off to London again on the train. He rang later, saying, 'You look more like Sinead O'Connor than Paul.'

I said to Kerry, who came over for the day, 'I've shaved all my hair off but don't ask to see it, I'm not a circus freak,' then proceeded to take my wig off to show her. She said, 'Oh my God, it just makes you look more beautiful.' Come again, Kerry! She also said that it accentuated all my features and if it was her she'd be very happy with it. Ah, she has a knack of always saying the right thing.

I drank almost a bottle of wine by myself last night and am suffering this morning. I am hardly drinking at all, but now and again the old me says, 'Fuck it,' and I spend the rest of the day beating myself up because I have breast cancer and I am alive, and lots of women are dead and if they had the choice of living or giving up alcohol, I can guess what they might choose. I feel selfish for tempting the wrath of someone to stamp on my head and bring back my cancer, and I think about Mr Monypenny and Helen and Gill Donovan at Velindre and how fantastic they have been to me, and what they would think of me knocking back the wine when they are going out of their way to save my life.

November 15, Wednesday

Cathy was very nice and reminded me a bit of Babs. She was so laid back about it all, but I am an obsessive information-gatherer. She is having another lumpectomy and her nodes removed. Her lump is smaller than mine. I asked if they knew that the cancer had spread to the lymph nodes and she said they were taking them out as a precaution. I showed her my book on nutrition and the one by Dr Susan Love, and said they had been really useful to me but that some people were not information gatherers, so that was fine if she thought they might be too much info. I don't know, maybe it's better to be that way; she was very stoical about it all. I wondered if she ever sank a bottle of wine over this, or was it just me, but didn't like to ask. I also wondered did she ever stay awake at night and worry if she would make it to sixty, but I didn't like to ask that either. She has to have chemo this time.

November 16, Thursday

My fertility is all up the spout. I had a period after my last chemo session and it stopped, then it comes back again in dribs and drabs. Maybe this is a good sign that my ovaries are giving up the ghost. After all, they are my oestrogen-producing monsters. Having said that, it could mean that I am propelled into an early menopause, which is OK as I don't want my ovaries. But I know from my mother and Rhodri's mother that it's hot flushes, irritability, mood swings and sleepless nights. Oh well, then I won't be able to tell the difference between the menopausal me and the pre-menopausal me.

November 17, Friday

No Welsh today. I had to stay in for a delivery of a desk from MFI to put some order into the chaos that is my middle room. It's a nice desk which is much better-looking than the previous one, but I really wish I had a spare room to put it in. Even though my rooms are IKEA's open-plan dream, it would be nice to shut the door on them sometimes and not have to worry about the mess.

Alison K came over with Erin and I told Erin (18 months) to look and learn but, if there was ever a man around, to pretend she didn't have a clue. Alison K did not approve, and I told her I had made a rod for my own back over the years being an ardent bloody feminist, and it just meant every flat-pack bit of furniture (which, let's face it, is almost every bit of furniture these days) I've had to put together because Rhodri is a sensitive new man and because of this feels he can be excused for not knowing how to do these things. There was a time when *I* didn't know how to do these things, I just looked at the bit of paper like everyone else. I told Alison K this and she said, 'Oh, he's a creative.' Hmm.

November 18, Saturday

It's been raining for days; it's driving me a bit mad. My mother offered to take the children but I thought I would save it for when I need it most after next week. So Rhodri is working all weekend and I have them to myself – lucky me. Julia came down for a flying visit and we just watched telly all day with the children jumping over the furniture and throwing cushions at each other with nothing much else to do other than destroy the house.

November 19, Sunday

Rhodri is working almost every weekend up until Christmas. He really has no idea how hard it is for me, emotionally if nothing else, to have to deal with going to chemo and him not being around. 'Get someone to stay with you,' he says, not thinking that completely disrupts their lives and they have children too (Julia and Jo). To be honest I feel sometimes it's easier to be on your own because when people are here, we don't have a spare room and it's a hassle. Anyway, I have my student, Rachel, who I agreed to have assigned to me to follow my treatment, coming to the chemo session next Wednesday, which Rhodri was more than eager to get out of, and will think about asking someone to come and stay over on Wednesday night after the chemo.

This morning I took the boys to Merlin's Castle, a nearby indoor play place, with the intention of letting them rush around like mad things on castles, slides, etc. while I drank cappuccino and read the paper. As per bloody usual the reality was somewhat different. I ordered lunch when I got there for us all and they were running about – fine so far, then lunch came, sausage and chips for them, soup for me. Osian managed to tip an entire bottle of water over Elis who was so wet, I had to wring his clothes out, and Elis said he wanted to go home. Then they started singing Happy Birthday over a Tannoy to some child who was having a birthday party, and Osian started crying, saying it was too noisy and he wanted to go home now. All this after I'd spent well over £16 and only had my arse on a seat for less than half an hour. I got them both to eat their food, told Elis to run around and his clothes would dry and sat Osian on my lap for an hour and a half while I drank my coffee and read the paper with him intermittently saying, 'I need to go home now.'

I took Elis to the *Dr Who* concert down in the Bay –

Rhodri was directing. Hazel has come to look after Osh, which I thought might be a bit of a nightmare as he is so mummy mummy at the moment and doesn't sleep unless I put him to bed. But I figure Hazel is a trained nursery professional (she's from Osh's crèche) and is experienced enough to put up with a bit of hassle. When I left them they were sat on the sofa under a blanket eating liquorice laces and Osh didn't even notice I'd gone. We arrived at the Millennium Stadium and there was some confusion over our seats and we had to move and were sitting behind the First Minister, Rhodri Morgan. Elis is always asking me who is the boss of Wales, so I said, 'See that man in front? HE is the boss of Wales – his name is Rhodri Morgan.'

'So two Rhodris,' Elis said 'are the boss tonight. Daddy is the boss of this show and he is the boss of Wales.'

The concert was absolutely fab. There were Daleks and monsters and Cyber-men coming from all over the place. *Dr Who* (who is actually David Tennent) was running the show and the orchestra played tracks from the series. Elis was spellbound by it all and halfway through he turned to me and said, 'I just can't believe this.'

'What?' I said, thinking he was going to say, 'I've seen *Dr Who*,' and he said, 'I'm sat behind the boss of Wales.' Oh, he's definitely going to be a politician. We went to the scanner around the back of the Millennium Centre after the show to see Rhodri, and Elis sat in the scanner and said he wanted to be a director when he grew up. Ho hum, popstardom and riches out of the window then, for now.

November 20, Monday

Martyn came over today to discuss my return to work. I had emailed him and said I wanted to come back, all being well, in June and then have a staggered return. He said it was all fine and I would have to see the BBC doctor before I returned to make sure I was fit enough. I wondered if it was Dr Who, but apparently it's someone in BUPA. He brought two Advent calendars and cakes for the boys – very sweet of him. Kerry came over and we looked at a house. She has decided she is definitely moving to the Cardiff area now. Hurrah! I knew I would eventually wear her down. The house was on an estate; it was big, but not very nice and very expensive. It would need a lot of money to bring it up to date but it did have loads of rooms. Thankfully, she didn't like it so we came back and looked some more up on the internet which were more suitable. She's coming back Wednesday to have a look.

November 21, Tuesday

Went to get my bloods checked at the hospital this morning and my white cell count was borderline. I missed an acupuncture session last week and I think this could have some bearing on it. I have to go back tomorrow to get my blood done again. They think it will be up by the morning and that the third chemo will be able to go ahead.

I so want to get the session over with, number three coming up, but I am beginning to dread having to go to the hospital. They are all really, really nice but I am getting a needle aversion for one thing, and I just don't want to be there. Rhodri isn't coming to chemo with me, he's finishing early so he can look after the children.

November 22, Wednesday

I was dreading going to the hospital and don't think I'll come on my own again, although I'm meeting my student Rachel so I'm not on my own really. I'm beginning to wish I didn't have the student and haven't actually done anything with her yet, but she's got to learn from someone and why not someone like me, who doesn't stop talking. Am reading *The Ten-Minute Life Coach*, which has taken over from *The Tibetan Book of Living and Dying*. It's fundamentally Buddhist in its ethos but a bit snappier, although I will return to *Tibet* when I get a minute. Anyway, it's about talking yourself up and NEVER being disparaging about yourself, so I'm trying to hold this in my mind. Rachel is lucky to have me, I think.

I was driving reluctantly towards the hospital, and I looked up and there was an enormous rainbow over the entire place and I was reminded of Rhodri's Auntie Sally's card to me, which made me cry when I got it, as she has also been ill. She had written *Behind every cloud there's always sunshine* and it gave me a big smile and a bit of a kick up the arse for being so miserable.

Had to wait in the hospital for three hours, which isn't long in total, but last time it was only an hour. The good news was that my blood was up, so I had the chemo. Rachel is very nice and very young; I chatted away, filling silences with just about everything. Not sure I can keep that up for the next three sessions. I told her I thought cancer was life-affirming and I saw it as a positive thing, and she said she was surprised by that, which I was surprised about, then I realised she's in her twenties so why would she think she was ever going to die? In fact, most people at forty don't think they are going to die either, I guess.

I hate the drips, I hate the smell, I hate trying to be happy and bright when I just want to get out of there.

When I came home, Kerry was there with Daisy and she left her while she went to see a house, looking very liberated. Julia and Pip arrived at the same time and took it in turns holding baby Daisy so I had a full house.

Julia had been to have a mammogram at BUPA and will get the results next week. I'm sure it will all be fine but we all do need to check. Chemo started to take effect late afternoon and I was very tired by the time Rhodri came back with the children at six. I couldn't keep my eyes open and had to go to bed where I stayed all night.

November 23, Thursday

Ian P from work emailed me to ask how I was and as he did, I was sobbing at my computer. I am feeling really low today. I am convinced it's the lack of acupuncture – I must have two sessions in between chemo, in future. I decided to ring the counsellor from the BBC helpline as I think I might need someone to help me along. *Ten-Minute Life Coach* says don't be afraid to buy in help, so I thought the counsellor would be just what I need right now. Told Ian P I was a bit down in the dumps and he is coming over next Wednesday to take me to the sea and buy me chips – sounds just the thing. 'Taking my devils for an airing' as Dylan Thomas would say.

I am beginning to feel stir crazy at home, and the thought of going back to work is not as scary as it has been. I need structure and a bit of purpose, as long as it's for only four days a week.

I must start going out for some walks. I don't seem to leave the house much and have stopped shopping now for the sake of my bank balance, so I will endeavour to have a walk every day. The weather is so wet and cold here though. It's been raining for days.

Julia came down today to take Osh up to the farm. Rhodri is working late tonight and Friday. Elis is OK, you can stick him in front of the telly, but Osh is higher maintenance and this time around after chemotherapy I feel so tired I can hardly stay awake. Have just been lying on the sofa all day watching telly and dozing, which is fine – can't really do much else. Spent the evening with Elis on Playstation and me lying in his bunk, watching him play. I found it difficult to get up and he went to bed at eight, so did I. I am completely exhausted.

November 24, Friday

Alexander Litvinenko, a former Russian spy, has been poisoned with radiation and has died. Elis came downstairs this morning while I was reading about it on the BBC news website and asked me why he died. I said he had been a spy and someone poisoned him, and as I was talking about it, it came on Sky News and he said, 'My God, it's on the news too.'

Him wanting to be a spy and all, this really caught his imagination. They were explaining on the telly in graphic detail how radiation kills you. Basically it kills the fast dividing cells and eventually will shut down your vital organs. I know chemo is a very controlled version of this but it's a little close to home for me at the moment and got me to thinking about my vital organs and why the bloody hell no one was checking those.

Gill Donovan's colleague, Lizzie, rang me from the hospital. They'd run a check on the supplements I am taking and have advised me not to take anything during chemo because they are antioxidants and therefore protecting cells they want to kill. Great. I've already been taking them during three sessions so now I'll be obsessing for the rest of my life over it. Still, if nothing else, it's got me off my arse, juicing again and eating satsumas like they were chocolates. I said I was worried that I'd pick up bugs and colds off the children, and was convinced the high dosages in the supplements were protecting me. She said that wouldn't put them off, giving me the chemo, the white blood cell count was the important thing. I will do as she says.

I asked her about radiotherapy, thinking it might make

me feel sick and I'd have to have needles, but she said it would be a walk in the park compared to chemo. I wouldn't feel sick, and it would take me longer to get dressed and undressed than have it. It is only for four weeks, not six, so that's good news too, so only three chemo sessions, which are the bits I don't like, to get through.

I asked about my hair growing back during radiotherapy. She said it would come back after the fifth session but a bit like baby hair – although it's growing back already. Then I said, 'And now a rather big question. How do you know that the cancer hasn't spread to my vital organs?' She said they could never tell me 100 per cent I was cured but the surgeon was pleased with my tumour removal and all the steps they are taking now – the chemo, radio and Tamoxifen – are curative; they are steps to cure me of cancer.

Every time they take my blood samples my vital organs are checked, kidney and liver. If there were any abnormalities, they would let me know. I am in a system where I am checked constantly and will have yearly mammograms and come to the clinic every year. If I ever want to ring them during those times, I will have instant referral. So I did feel better after that. It's like Lizzie said, the further away from diagnosis, the easier it is to come to terms with it, which I know will be the case.

They are amazing, Gill and Lizzie and the people at Cancer Care Cymru. They are not the NHS, they are a charity and they work alongside the NHS. If they weren't there, I wonder who would I pick the phone up to call and ask the questions that haunt me; sometimes for days. They answer you, just like that, and don't think you are mad asking them. I do have Helen, of course, but Gill is in the thick of it, going through it with me, I feel. I am so lucky because I have a big support network. I said this to Gill and she said she was talking to a lady on the phone who is in her seventies going through chemotherapy and doesn't have any family, and it just makes me feel so blessed that I am supported by people I love and who love me.

I asked Gill how she does it – deals with sick people, some very sick, all the time, and she said, 'It is a privilege to work with you all.' I told her *we* were the privileged ones.

Rhodri came home at eight with a Chinese. Julia has taken Elis up to the farm for the weekend so we watched two episodes of *Lost* and it was really nice to be together.

November 25, Saturday

I still feel as if I should be in a retirement home, kipping my life away, I am so tired. Would I actually enjoy doing that? When the to-do lists get done by someone else, when I have stopped obsessing about my future, and will be in it, what will have happened? Where will my children be, where will my husband be, will we be kipping pensioners together? How will I feel when I don't have to worry about rice or turkey for Christmas, about whether the goldfish can go another day and live without me cleaning them, without children's birthday parties and school fetes to occupy my time? How will I feel when it all stops and I have nothing to do except the one thing I so want to do which has eluded me all week, which is sleep. Pretty fucking bored, I imagine – let's hope telly improves before that all kicks in. I owe it to the world of media to return to try and get some decent programmes made.

Went to Ian J's tonight. Ah, the upside of chemotherapy – you don't want to drink. I know, I can't actually believe I have written those words. You drive to someone's house, eat their food, enjoy a short burst of their charming company and leave about 10.30 – job done, catch up, nice food, no hangover, no staying up until three in the morning. Rhodri on the other hand did stay until three in the morning and woke me up when he came in; I then spent an hour and a half awake. I am no longer getting up in the night as I used to. I was getting up for two hours in the night, but ended up all cold and uncomfortable on the sofa watching an episode of *Midsomer Murders* or something, when I already knew who'd done it. The children are still having a whale of a time at my parents' farm, so no worries there. Whatever would I do without my wonderful parents?

November 26, Sunday

I woke very early again and made Beef Bourguignon for tea and an enormous veggie chilli for the freezer – just call me Delia. Have a bit of a spring in my step now that chemo is disappearing into the horizon.

Went to see the new Bond film with Rhodri and Ian J. That Daniel Craig is eminently shaggable! God, I'd so do him. Can't imagine he's going to be wandering up my street sometime soon, though. If he does, though, we couldn't do it in the marital bed – that would be sacrilege, PLUS the bedroom is a dumping ground for all 'pending' washing and ironing so it's never properly tidy and I'd have to tidy up anyway if he knocked on the door – so we'd have to find somewhere else to do it. That would all start getting a bit awkward then – what was I doing in such and such hotel and why wasn't I answering my mobile . . . I can see my affair with Daniel Craig might not be as straightforward as I first thought.

Osh and Elis came back, filling the house with their babble and chatter and treading potato into the carpet. Osh seems to come on about six months every time he goes to stay with my parents. He said, very matter-of-factly, that, 'Dinosaurs eat grass.' Lloyd is obsessed with dinosaurs, so Osh is getting into them too and he's just like a little boy with opinions and singing songs – they had a great time.

I had one of those nice kicks up the arse that I need when I start to feel a little bit sorry for poor old cancer victim me. I was reading the *Sunday Mirror*, which is my paper of choice these days, since it takes less than half an hour to read, tells me all I need to know in a nutshell and I don't have to sift through reams and reams of rainforest on a Sunday just because I purport to be middle-class.

What I have found in life is that if you surround yourself with like-minded people, which we all do as we all wish to see ourselves reflected in our friends, they will invariably give you the opinions, reviews and hot topics of the week from the news. This saves the price of an expensive Sunday newspaper and also allows me to read about the exploits of the latest *I'm A Celebrity* in the *Sunday Mirror*, safe in the knowledge that by the following weekend I will have assumed all their opinions, my friends' that is, not the *Sunday Mirror*'s, and pass them off as my own.

Anyway, there was an article in it about a little girl with leukaemia which I would normally ignore, not because I am a heartless callous bitch, but because the thought of any child suffering is too much to bear. Even Rhodri turns the news over temporarily if there are bad news children stories now. I know it's cowardly but I think it's a parent's way of trying to live with the 'my child might die' scenario which sometimes haunts us all.

This little girl was keeping a blog of her treatment and quite honestly I was ashamed of my whimpering about a bloody needle in my arm and going on how the veins in my arm hurt and how I think one of them has collapsed, and about the smell of the hospital and the place. And this child was a happy smiling cherub who I wanted to put in a bubble and protect against the chemo which was relentless for her, and she had to have deep injections into her beautiful fragile little body. She served to remind me that I should be grateful for the life that I am living, for my second chance and, as Maya Angelou put it, 'Just because I am in pain it doesn't mean I have to become one.'

I am sending a wish to Santa and Buddha and Jesus and Mohammed to look after that little angel – please.

November 27, Monday

Another sleepless night. However, my sleeplessness is exacerbated by the start of the Ashes, and there have been some ground rules laid down for the gentlemen in this house. Rhodri waits until twelve at night to see the Ashes start; he takes a duvet and pillows downstairs so he can lie on the sofa and sleep in between the boring bits (isn't that all of it?), then when he realises that he has to get up at 7.30, and probably do a fourteen-hour day, as he has of late, he decides to come to bed. This is any time between one and four o'clock in the morning – about the time I have nicely drifted off into my cocoon.

He did this last night when I had deliberately not gone to bed until twelve so that I could get a stab at an eight-hour sleep. I immediately awoke as he was shuffling round the bedroom turning the heating off and pulling the duvet I had been sleeping under right over to his side. Anyway, I went mad saying he was bloody selfish and that it was bad enough that I could only sleep for five to six hours a night without him waltzing in the bedroom when he felt like it, and if he wanted to watch the Ashes he was to either sleep in the bunks (which he hates as they are too small) or stay on the sofa. He was under no circumstances to come back to our room and disturb me – so there. This is the point in my life when I wish we had bought a brand new house with en suite and four bedrooms for a cheaper price than our three up, two down, fur coat, no knickers Llandaff house. Then we'd have a spare room. I ended up going to sleep in the bunk, which was fine, but woke up about six which meant I only got about five and a half hours' sleep. I think

I'm getting less sleep than Alison W next door and she has a new baby. Still, I will stop obsessing about it. It's not as if I've got a top job in the city to go to, is it?

I got my own back on Rhodri this morning – not, of course, that marriage is an ongoing set of one-upmanship. I woke about 6.15 in the bottom bunk 'snug as a bug in a rug', went into our bedroom to get a cardigan and slippers to go and have a nice cup of tea, and by accident stood on the 'First Christmas' book, which peeled out a verse of 'Away in a Manger' very loudly and woke Rhodri up with an enormous start. Sitting bolt upright in bed as if he had been electrocuted, he said in his sleep-induced haze, 'I AM being nice to you.' Obviously he had been dreaming about NOT being nice to me.

November 28, Tuesday

Until you cannot have children you do not realise what an utterly crass and deeply personal question it is to ask someone, 'Are you having any more?' It's not that I mind *not* being able to have any more children – I am nearly forty, for God's sake. I have two very healthy children and thank God for that every day. But as the same God is my witness, I will never ask anyone that question again. Rachel, my student, and one of my neighbours both asked me this week if I wanted more children. Are these people mad! I have had breast cancer, I am having chemotherapy – five months ago I thought I might actually die. Why would I even dream of bringing any more children, even if I could, into that uncertain world? Are you fucking bonkers?

Made an appointment with the brain woman Deborah for next Wednesday. Now I've had my kick up the arse from the angel in the paper, I'm not sure I need someone to pull me through, am not sure what she can help me with – but I bet every nutter who goes in there (like me) thinks they are the sanest, most rational person on the planet. I keep putting it off, thinking I'll have it after chemo, or after all my treatment, but as work will pay for my sessions I might as well go now, when I am in the thick of it all. Went to Welsh class – still very confusing, definitely a longterm project.

November 29, Wednesday

I had lunch with Ian P, went to an absolutely fab pub, the Plough and Harrow. Firstly we had a little walk along the coastal path. Ian P is so sweet. He and his girlfriend are splitting up and I've always thought that he and Kate would make a lovely couple. I showed him a picture of her which I had on my phone and he said she looked very nice. Texted Kate and said I know she liked Mark but Ian P was lovely and available and thought she looked nice. I have not heard back from her which means she is either a) mortally offended or b) just too busy to respond. Must call her soon. My quest to find a wife for the two Ians in my life continues.

Went to the shops for a Welsh-language birthday card for Rhodri's mother and to IKEA for two frames to put photos of Osh and Elis in for her sixtieth birthday. We have got this present called 'In the Paper' and it's a spoof Flintshire evening paper with a funny bit about Rhodri's mother being sixty on the front page and a photo of her when she was a baby. It's all good fun, and the family have also all pooled together to buy her a digital camera.

We're all booked in to the Cawdor Hotel in Llandeilo: Sioned and Ali, Owain and Eva, Branwen, Patrick and Cari Mair, Ela, me, Rhodri, Osh and Elis with Rhodri's parents. I'm sure it will be lovely. The hotel is really nice. Rhodri and I went there just before my diagnosis without the children.

I said to Rhodri, 'The last time we were in that hotel I

didn't have cancer,' and he replied, 'You did have cancer, you just didn't know about it.' Pedant. Anyway, the last time Rhodri and I were there about seven months ago, we were shagging like rabbits. I'm not sure we will have the opportunity with two children cramping our style.

I have no idea if my period is due. I was supposed to be keeping a note to see if my periods had stopped because of the chemo, but I was eating chocolate biscuits earlier which is a sure sign that my period is on its way. Damn. What's the point of being in a hotel with your husband if you can't shag him, and hotel sex is so much better than sex at home, where 500 other things are running around in your head – ooh, that pile of washing needs to be put out and ooh, those sheets haven't been changed for a fortnight and ooh, it's so late I really need to sleep. Whereas when you're in a hotel those thoughts don't really pop into your head (or if they do that's very sad) and there's something quite sleazy about having lots of sex in a hotel room (well, OK, managing to do it twice). Sex has taken a back seat in our lives at the moment.

November 30, Thursday

What do I do with my days? I don't know, but I never seem to sit down for more than two minutes. I went to see Rosie today and told her I thought that my chemo was worse because I didn't have acupuncture the week before; so she has rung around because she is away next week and I am going to see a friend of hers, who coincidentally is in Penarth, not far from the brain woman, so I'll have a Penarth sort of a day.

Rhodri has gone to his cricket dinner in the village. He came in tonight and we were chatting and he goes, 'Is this a good time to have an awkward conversation?' I fucking *hate* it when he starts any conversation like that because I automatically think he is shagging someone else, or has cancer (I beat him to that one), or something else terrible is wrong – and I get so angry when he follows this opening question with something completely banal.

More often than not, he tells me that he has to go away to work on a project, and sure enough, he's asking my permission to do the Kirov Ballet, which is great, but will take him away, although he'll be back on my birthday.

Will I let him do it? It's his job, for heaven's sake! Am I going to say, 'No, you can't,' when it's his job that keeps the roof over our heads? And even if he did have a choice, which I am sure he does, am I, the wicked witch of the west, going to say, 'No, actually you can't do that.'

'I thought you and the children could come up to London,' he said. I don't want to go to London for my fortieth birthday. I am thanking the bloody Lord I am fucking alive to see my fortieth birthday. Why would I want to spend it in a hotel room in London when I can be around my friends and family in my own safe little house? Plus I know my chemo is supposed to finish by then but it might not; there might be a blip and I can't make any plans, he just doesn't fucking get it.

So then I had a go at him for not getting it, saying that his life had not changed at all except perhaps it had become easier because I was home all the time, whereas mine had changed fundamentally and he had never once said I was doing great. And he said, 'I just told Pip you were doing great now on the phone while you were upstairs' and, like yeah, that's supposed to make me feel better?

'How am I supposed to know what you say to other people?' I ranted.

'You *are* doing great,' he said. 'There, I just told you.'

'Yes, but I practically put the words in your mouth,' I snarled, 'so it doesn't count.'

Then I'm thinking I should change my single therapy session to marriage guidance sessions. As soon as chemo is

133

over I will be getting onto a bloody counsellor to show Rhodri what a complete and utter selfish bastard he is.

December 1, Friday

Tomorrow's today! Those were the words Elis screamed from his darkened room this morning. It's the first of December – COUNTDOWN TO CHRISTMAS. We have six Advent calendars in our house, three for Elis and three for Osh. Elis woke Osh up by turning his light on and thrusting a sweet into his mouth, which he promptly spat out, saying, 'Don't want it.' He didn't want the two chocolates from his other Advent calendars either, which left me no option but to eat them myself.

After an entire year of waiting, Christmas is well and truly on its way. I banned Elis from talking about Christmas in about February because I couldn't stand an entire year of it. I lament the loss of Christmas so much myself; I don't want it to be over. I think what I like about it so much is that all the family are together and it's a two-week holiday where it's OK to stay in the house and not do much, which is what I like doing best. There's no large itinerary planned out for the day before you even open your eyes, no agenda to be up at seven and off by nine, just leisurely long mornings spent in your pyjamas and not bothering to bath the children and letting them eat as much crap as they like because it's Christmas.

Even Rhodri subscribes to the 'must have a rest at Christmas' philosophy. Last year he didn't have much of an option as he was in bed with a bad back for most of the holiday.

The previous year we had stayed at my parents' – in bunk beds – and he was on top (as it were). In his haste to get down to see the children's faces when they saw their presents, he fell out of the top bunk and broke two of his ribs. He didn't tell anyone about it for days because 'he didn't want to make a fuss'! I'm hoping this year he will actually be able to get out of bed on a voluntary basis.

Elis still thinks that twenty-five days is too long to wait until Christmas. Last year around about this time he was very tired one night and was crying, which is very much out of character as he rarely cries, and when he does you know it's something serious, and I said, 'What's wrong?' He said, 'It's just Christmas – it's so long to wait,' and I said, 'But you've got your calendar now and you're counting down.' And he said, 'Have you seen how many chocolates are on that calendar? It'll take for ever.'

Oh, how I wish twenty-five days were a lifetime to me. But I suppose they could be. Why not turn time on its head and instead of thinking about it as time running out and life being short, I could be like my darling Elis and view time in all its fabulous glory. Twenty-five wonderful days to have to wait, each one of them as special as the next.

Instead of wishing my chemo were over and my radiotherapy were over and that we were going on holiday and thinking that I'd have to start work and how will I live with the threat of cancer returning and how would I face that again and wishing away months and years of my entire life . . . I could spend my time just being in it, just savouring each precious moment. Every time tomorrow is today I will resolve to do that.

December 2, Saturday

In Llanelli at the Cawdor Hotel for Rhodri's mother's sixtieth birthday. Hotel lovely, food lovely, company lovely. Rhodri had to stay with Osh until nine as he wouldn't sleep but eventually he went off. No possibility of having hotel sex as all in the same room. Me, Rhodri and the children that is, not the entire family.

December 3, Sunday

I feel a little bit hungover today after the meal last night. Rhodri and I were the last men standing. I had a terrible night's sleep. I could kill Rhodri sometimes. It was blowing a gale outside so it was difficult to sleep anyway, PLUS, twice in the middle of the night Rhodri turned the telly on to see the score in the Ashes. We had been unable to find the remote control so both times it came on at full volume, waking me up with such a start I thought someone had died, and waking Osh up into the bargain. It had me saying very loudly, 'Turn that fucking telly off NOW.' He's mental.

We had lunch in a really nice restaurant nearby but Osh wouldn't sit down; he was running around and some old bags upstairs complained about the children. My attitude was, 'Fuck them'. The kids weren't being badly behaved, they were just being children.

Then a woman asked me if the children could avoid eating dessert on their leather sofas as they were very expensive and would have to be recovered if they got ice cream on them. Suddenly the working-class chip on my shoulder was prompting me to say: 'I know how much leather sofas cost – mine was shipped over from Italy, you stupid bitch, and if they get any ice cream on them I'll give you a packet of wet wipes to bloody well clean it off, just as I do with mine.'

But instead I said, 'At the table, children,' to Cari and Elis and sat there and ate my ice cream. Then I looked and saw that Osh's arm was completely covered in chocolate mousse and he had been rolling it all over the 'very expensive' leather sofa, so I did have to get out my wet wipes and give it a once-over when the snooty cow was not looking. Came up a treat, it did.

December 4, Monday

I slept for ten and a half hours last night. It was bloody heaven. I cannot remember when I last slept that long. I lay on our bed with Osh because he was refusing to go off to sleep and was stood in his cot shouting, 'Mummy, I want to come out!' at the top of his voice. It was about 8.30 and before I knew it, it was an hour later, Rhodri was taking Osh to his cot and I cleaned my teeth and just stayed there all night without waking once. The heating coming on at seven, as opposed to six, when it had been waking me, is working because I don't wake until seven now. So I feel great for the sleep. As predicted though, coming off my supplements I have snivels immediately, a bit of a runny nose and a tight chest with a cough. I am willing my white blood cells to hang in there and keep up their spirits. I visualise them as little soldiers fighting the good fight against everything that is thrown at them, the poor buggers – like that battle scene in *The Lord of the Rings* when you think, Bloody hell, they are so not going to win this, they are completely outnumbered – and everything that could be hurled at them is, but they win.

Saw Kylie on Sky News entertainment – God, she looks fantastic and a bit of weight really suits her. Well, weight in Kylie's terms is slightly different to weight in my terms. I would be very happy with her hair. I wonder what the texture will be, as they say it can be different from before. Maybe instead of being curly it will be straight and sleek, and I will be dyeing it this fab red colour that is my wig.

I quite like the idea of very short hair and think that when it grows back I won't be as obsessed with it looking perfect as I was before. Much as I love my wig, and it has really made me feel great about myself at a time when I really need it, I will be glad to get my own hair back.

Four days into December and I have broken open one of Osh's Advent calendars and eaten the rest of the chocolates.

I thought, I'll only have one, so opened the 5th, then thought, Fuck it, they have four calendars, since Sioned gave them another one at the weekend. I think she must have forgotten she had already given them one. And Osh is only two, so he doesn't know what time of day it is and my need is greater than his. Ooh, am feeling a bit guilty about eating them now, and a bit sick.

I am scrubbing the interior of the fireplace. No, I haven't gone completely obsessive compulsive; I'm having a multifuel burner fitted so this is the last chance to get rid of dirt on the bricks. It's hard work, I bet Rhodri will not even notice.

The CD on the computer is broken and it's Rhodri's lifeline, as he downloads stuff on to his Ipod for work. He was his usual ineffectual, 'So what are we going to do?' meaning, 'What are YOU going to do?' And I went into my usual defensive mode: 'What do *you* think WE should do?' and, 'We are not buying a new one, as we don't have any money, so what are you going to do?' And he said, 'I'm working full time.'

'Oh,' I said, 'I wish I was working full time,' when actually I don't, and then I said, 'OK, I'll get it fixed,' because he's right, I am here at home all day. It's just that I resent doing everything, and even if I was working full time he would still expect me to do it. The other day I asked him how we are going to manage with the cleaning and the ironing when I go back to work. My mother and Joanne – Kim and Aggie as I call them – have been coming down every other week at the moment and doing it for me. Instead of saying we'd do it together, a bit at a time, he said, 'I'll pay for a cleaner,' because the truth is, it would never occur to him to clean anything unless he was instructed to do so by me. To the best of my knowledge, in the ten years I have known him he has never cleaned a toilet. How he thinks it gets clean, I don't know. In fact, I wonder how long it would take for him to notice it needed cleaning. If I didn't have children I would conduct an experiment. PLUS he says, 'I'll pay for a cleaner,' like spending £100 a month on someone coming to our house is his decision and I have no say in how HIS money should be spent.

I've opened an account for bills as we have never had a joint bank account. The other day I sat down and worked out how much of my money goes out on household expenses and food, and the result is: every single penny. There is NO disposable income, so no wonder I have been overdrawn for years. I am waiting to do an audit of Rhodri's expenditure when his next statement comes through. He didn't seem to think the joint bills account was a good idea – no, I bet he doesn't. The truth will all be revealed shortly.

Blowing an absolute gale here today. It's definitely time for wood-burning stoves.

December 5, Tuesday

Christmas will be coming much earlier to this house than to the rest of the country. I consume whole Advent calendars in one sitting. Osh is taking random sweets and chocolates out of his three and Elis religiously does it every day but somehow is already on the sixth of December. In my experience of these things he'll forget a couple of days and hopefully Christmas will come on Christmas Day.

Went to Welsh today then came home and made an aubergine casserole for later (just call me Jamie) and picked both Elis and Osh up to get a Christmas tree. I had both of them, two reindeer Christmas tree decorations which Elis wanted and a five foot Christmas tree in my shopping trolley and they all fitted. I don't know why I am so surprised. I usually manage to cram about one hundred and twenty pounds' worth of food in one in Tescos and that never looks like anything and never lasts more than a week.

Buying a tree reminds me of one of the worst rows Rhodri and I ever had. It was two years ago (not that I bear a grudge), the first Christmas in this house and, although the house was a mess, I wanted it to be really special as it was Osh's first Christmas. So I went shopping with my mother and bought a tree and when I told Rhodri the tree cost twenty pounds, he went mad. I said, 'What century are you living in?' and I went on about how he was a miserable git and that Christmas was all about families and being together, and even though the house was a mess it was special for the children and they don't see the mess or remember the mess but they do see and remember that their mum went out and got them a tree. I was so angry that I didn't speak to him for about two days and I never do that.

If ever I have a row, within a short space of time I have to clear the air. The only other time I have not spoken to him for a few days was when he cheated at Scrabble. He is a Scrabble fanatic and I was winning, I was bloody winning and I am crap at it – he's read books on it and has studied the Scrabble dictionary, he is a Scrabble geek, basically, and he couldn't stand it because I was winning. He cheated by not going and changing all his counters, as he knew that I would have them when it was my turn and that I wouldn't be able to go as he couldn't. I know technically it's in the rules, but he could not stand the thought that I might actually beat him at his precious game. I have not played Scrabble with him again, except once when he was ill, and I felt sorry for him and he spoke to me as if I was a little girl saying, 'Now, Shell, do you know what I would do if I were you?' 'Fuck off,' I wanted to say, but I humoured him because he is a man and that is what we women do.

Anyway, I digress with this Scrabble talk. So the upshot of 'The Christmas Tree Incident' as I refer to it, is that every time I so much as mention him buying, or should I say paying for, a Christmas tree as it would never occur to

140

him to actually go and buy a Christmas tree, he says, 'Yes, of course, no problem,' and smiles, knowing that if he dared to mention the cost or that it's bad for the environment I would shove the bloody tree down his Grinch-like throat.

I didn't get the tree out of the car as it was too wet, and by the time Rhodri came back, it was too late to decorate it. I had lost a little of my Christmas cheer because I slept badly and am tired and think I might have a chest infection, so need to get myself checked out with the doctor tomorrow. I'll save tree-decorating for the morning, when I shall be as bright and cheery as one of Santa's little helpers.

Brain ironing woman tomorrow – I'm having major second thoughts about her. I am sure she is very nice, but I'm now thinking she might disrupt my positivity, as the Spice Girls would say. I don't want to be blubbing into a Kleenex in the office of some woman I've never met before. I might not go after this time. I was going to go into her office and say, 'I kept my appointment, but actually I don't want to come again.' But I will just see how it goes and if I feel OK about it.

Also I'm going to Rosie's friend, the acupuncturist near the brain ironer. Then I'm off to Clare's house in the evening for the works Christmas get-together. My day is like a bus, things always come in threes. It will be the first time I've seen a lot of them from work in months – feels very weird. I am Clare's secret Santa and I have got her a notepad which is entitled *Who's to Blame – why blame yourself when you can blame someone else*. It lists problems on the left and potential wrongdoers on the right and you connect them in the middle – before long you will be 'blame storming in no time!' I'm sure it will go down with great hilarity. I may get one for Rhodri, although he might start blaming me for everything then, instead of the other way round.

December 6, Wednesday

Rhodri was going into work late this morning, so he took the children to school and crèche then came back for breakfast. I was sawing bits off the Christmas tree to get it to fit in its holder and I roped him into doing it, and then I decorated it, and just before he left, he paused and said, 'It looks lovely,' and he meant it. It seems all the Whos down in Whoville have finally got to him.

I can't wait for Osh and Elis to get home and see it. I know Osh won't remember trees from previous years, so he will think it's magical. He's taken to saying 'Wow!' at everything exciting and new and I love that, that new pair of eyes to see something we have become blasé about or indifferent to. Life should be stuffed with a few more 'wows' about the everyday things we take for granted. I'm sat here looking at my beautiful Christmas tree thinking about my lovely children and husband and I feel like I am the luckiest person alive. Wow.

I went for acupuncture with Rosie's colleague. She was so nice and addressed my cold to get my chi flowing properly before she tackled my immune system. It was raining and pouring, as little Osh says, and the rain set off a car alarm and she told me about earthquakes in Uganda. When she was a little girl, she said, you knew an earthquake was coming because the shop alarms would go off. She also told me about her sister-in-law in India, who had breast cancer and was going through chemo. She went over and gave her sister-in-law a session. All very fascinating stuff – I felt like I knew her after an hour's session on her couch.

Then I had lunch and went to see my brain-ironer, Deborah. I am so in the wrong job! She has this bloody fab house decorated in Farrow and Ball paint (Chapel Green, same as my back door) and it was all quiet and calm and she works when she wants and clearly earns a lot of money doing this – unless, of course, she has a rich husband. I did say she had a lovely house but she did not respond, as I guess people like her do not wish to exchange small talk with us mad people.

I now want to be a counsellor and have a big house in Penarth and work when I want to, and pick the children up from school myself. I know I would be a good counsellor because all my friends use me as one anyway, so I would just be getting paid for what comes naturally. Bree and Kerry call me their guru on childrearing (my God, that's a scary thought) and my other friends are always after me for relationship advice. As I write this down now, I'm thinking, I'm not sure I am the correct person to be giving parenting or relationship advice, but there you go, that's what happens. PLUS, OF COURSE, I want to help people – or should I say, give people the tools to help themselves.

ANYWAY, never being one to need an excuse to talk, I basically talked at her for two hours; I couldn't believe the time because I thought, Oh my hour must be up now, and then realised I'd been there for two hours – she must have been reeling from it. I talked a lot about being a control freak and trying to turn my cancer into a positive rather than a negative.

She did very stereotypical counselling, nodding of the head, and occasionally saying, 'Yes,' and I thought, She's just playing a game and I'm doing all the work. I didn't think she would be of any use to me at all, because I've pretty much psycho-analysed myself to death. I told her I was in denial because I saw cancer patients in the hospital as sick people and didn't feel I was one of them, and that Rhodri was also in denial because he said we couldn't park in the spaces reserved for chemo patients and I had said, 'But I am a chemotherapy patient,' and that we had both laughed over our denial.

And I said I thought having cancer had made me re-evaluate my life and become a better parent, more tolerant and a better wife. I thought that my relationship with Rhodri was stronger; although we have issues, we certainly don't argue as much.

And I told her that I thought I was to blame for my cancer because I drank wine, and didn't breast feed and had children late in life and that was partly why I had really half-expected my diagnosis; and for years I had just been waiting for that day to arrive.

And I told her that I was afraid of dying and that even though I thought I couldn't live without my children, I knew that my children could live without me, but the thought of that was really more than I could bear, and then I started crying and I couldn't stop. I said that they were my entire life, and the thought of leaving them was the most painful thing of all: not the dying, or the cancer, but my children having to grow up without their mummy.

And I realised that being a jolly cancer victim is bloody hard work and sometimes you do need to talk to someone to tell them the things you are frightened to confront yourself, no matter how clued up you think you are, or how positive you are about everything in life.

My name is Michelle and I have cancer and I wish I didn't have it and I wish it was a bad dream and I wish it would go away.

And we talked about Rhodri and I told her that when I was diagnosed I wanted him to look after me, but he didn't really adopt that role. She said that if I acted all the time as if it wasn't a big deal (not her exact words but this is the gist) then how was he ever to know that I felt vulnerable and needed looking after?

And she asked me what he thought about my cancer, and I realised that in six months I had never once asked him, never once talked to him about it, not really, and that was a really major revelation for me.

How can I expect him to be this person I want him to be if I never tell him how I feel or ask his opinion? Although he can be a selfish bastard, Rhodri can also be insightful and supportive and a really good husband, and maybe I just don't give him the chance to be that. I realised that this had to change, it has to be different; this woman is giving me the tools and I need to use them. We have to talk about this.

Went to Clare's house for the office Christmas party. I had to be there by seven so I thought it might be a bit of a roll-on roll-off affair, processing us as quickly as possible, but it wasn't like that at all, it was really lovely. Clare and her partner Kevin are so welcoming and have such a gorgeous house.

I was very pissed by the end of it, despite my resolve not to drink much and was having a full-blown debate with Kevin over parenting programmes on television. They all said I looked great and it was really nice to see them all, and not at all daunting as I thought it might be. I'm hoping I wasn't too loud or overbearing and conversation-hogging, but suspect I might have been.

December 7, Thursday

We wish you a merry Christmas, we wish you a merry Christmas . . .

I have the hangover from hell. I am so not used to drinking now (hurrah, I love writing that) that, when I do, it really takes its toll.

Kerry came over and I said that every time I have a hangover she comes over so she must have a false impression of me, that I am always drinking. She has a goitre on her thyroid again and needs to have it drained. I am trying to convince her to go to an acupuncturist as the thyroid is tied into the immune system.

Sat down with Rhodri for supper tonight (still had a terrible headache) and I said that Deborah had pointed out that I never showed my vulnerability to him. I said I thought she was right and that we never really talked about

145

my cancer and I asked him what he thought about my illness. I felt quite awkward asking him, bizarrely, and this is what he said: 'Do you want me to tell you what I think you want to hear, or what I actually think?' Hm, OK, will deal with that later.

I said, 'I want you to tell me what you really think.' So he said, 'I think it is unfair that something like this happens to such a lovely person. I think there is a positive side to it though, that you have matured as a person and are very focused on the family, and my concern is that you will go back to your old ways,' meaning being a party girl who never actually goes to parties but drinks in the house, 'and you should try to hold on to all the positive things that have happened to you.'

So from his opening statement I am wondering if he edits the truth for me on a regular basis. He probably does. I felt uncomfortable with the bit about going back to my old ways, but he is only verbalising what I think in my own head: that I want to stay healthy and avoid alcohol as I know it's not good for me and it will definitely be 'high days and holidays only' drinking for me in the future.

I was glad I had asked him because it never occurred to me that he thought it was unfair that I should get it, and I thought that was a lovely thing to say as it came from the heart. It's not fair for *anyone* to get cancer, but I have it and I personally can't think that it's unfair because it's a fact and I have to deal with it. But it was nice to hear that from him, and I felt that maybe this was the start of something new between us.

December 8, Friday

Picked Elis up from school with Osh. We're going up to the farm tomorrow for the day to see Sarah, Fin and Diarmuid who are over from Ireland. Elis is very excited about seeing them. Managed to get them to bed early as they need lots of sleep to play with their cousins. Rhodri is still working horribly late; I'm really fed up with being on my own all the time.

December 9, Saturday

Took Osh for a walk to the Post Office to send a birthday present to baby Nancy, Ben and Brees' baby in Brighton. I'm hoping we can go and visit them in February, when Rhodri will have two weeks off. I went up to the farm to see Sarah. Julia was in bed all day with a hangover from her works party and Sarah, who is training to be a homeopath, had given her a remedy which gave her the runs. To which Sarah said, 'Yes, it does that sometimes, it's clearing out your system.' Julia looked like death when she got up.

Lloyd, Fin, Elis, Osh and Diarmuid were all running around the house like maniacs; God knows how she managed to sleep. As long as you can stay in bed though, when you feel like that, it's all that matters really.

I asked Diarmuid if he wanted a sleep-over and he did, so he and Elis watched *Star Wars* (the first movie). Osh was in bed. I had to keep telling them to be quiet because I wanted to watch it too; it's my favourite *Star Wars* film. Diarmuid wanted the light left on, which I did and then shut it off when I went to bed.

In the morning Elis came in and said Diarmuid was sick and had thrown up everywhere. He said, 'You didn't leave the light on, Shelley,' so I have probably traumatised him about sleeping at our house for evermore. Had to throw all the sheets, pillows and duvet out on the patio to deal with later, as I had to leave at nine to take them to the airport.

We were playing I Spy in the car on the way up to the farm; it was Diarmuid's turn and as he was about to I Spy he wound the window down, threw up, wound it back up again and said, 'I spy with my little eye something beginning with a.' I love children: when they are sick it is so perfunctory. Wind the window down, throw up, get on with life whereas us adults are groaning and moaning and have to go to bed immediately. Children have not grasped the concept of feeling sorry for themselves. I'm not sure when it comes.

I took them to the airport, had a Burger King and waved them off and came back. Elis got in the car and said, 'Ah, just me and you together. What shall we do? Have a chat?' I said, 'Yes, we'll have a chat.' I realised that I don't spend as much one-to-one time with him as I used to. Either Osh is about or we're in different rooms and I'm usually with Osh as he is the one you need to keep an eye on.

It's just with everything that has gone on over the last few months, life has been a bit chaotic. I will resolve to do more stuff with him, as what tends to happen is Osh stays with me and Rhodri does stuff with Elis.

Came home from the airport and did a mammoth washing of duvets and sheets. Osh was being a little devil and tipped two cups of orange juice on the sofa. I tapped him on the hand and said, 'Time out,' which is what they have in nursery if they are naughty, and he hit me back and said, 'No, you time out.' Obviously taking Top Tips in behaviour from his brother. So then I had to deal with the sofa, and by the time the boys went to bed there was bedding and cushions and sheets and duvets drying all over the house; the place was a mess and I didn't have the energy to do any more.

So I sat down feeling totally fed up that Rhodri was always working and I have to do everything, and I felt really angry with him and wanted to shout at him when he came in at nine. I was expecting him at eleven but he didn't go out with the presenters on the show, the main presenter broke his leg at the last minute so they have to get another one a short notice. They have been working late to get up to

148

speed on scripts etcetera. He brought some wine, so I had a glass.

He sat on the sofa and, instead of shouting that I was fed up with being on my own and him always working, I just started crying and said in a rational voice that I was fed up with being on my own all the time. It was hard work and I felt like a single parent, and the children were always asking where he was. He sat by me and put his arm around me but then I felt bad because I laid all that shit on him and there is nothing he can do about it, as that's his job.

So even though Deborah says to show I'm vulnerable, it sort of means you pass your shit on to someone else in some cases, and I didn't know if that was really going to make me better.

December 11, Monday

I mislaid my diary, which has my entire life in it, and thought I was due to see Deborah at 11.30, but was due at 10.15 so now I need a counsellor to counsel me for pissing off the counsellor. I turned up and said, 'Sorry if I'm early, I can come back,' to which she replied: 'No, you were due an hour ago.' So I had to trundle up to her room as if I was going to see the Headmistress and get her number for another appointment. I came back and still can't find my diary, despite tidying the house. I'm wondering if Osh has something to do with its disappearance.

I came back from Penarth and was looking out the window when a florist's van pulled up with a big bouquet of red roses for me. They were from Rhodri. Ah, complaining is now the new black.

I rang Kerry later and told her I had roses and that complaining was horrible as he couldn't do much about working late, and she said it was his job to listen to me moan and, even if he can't do much about it, he can show his support for me.

I will thank Deborah for pointing me in a direction I thought I didn't need to go in, namely opening up to my husband, and instead of thinking he's only interested in his own head, try to find out a little bit more about what is actually going on in it, rather than closing myself down to him.

December 12, Tuesday

Went to the hospital for a blood test. I only just scraped through, but the main thing was I can have chemo tomorrow. I was reading a breast helpline leaflet in the waiting room; it was rather fatalistic with regards to the possibility of having breast cancer twice, and more or less assumed it would happen. So I asked Gill about it, as I know of a few people who have had it twice and I'm now getting more paranoid than usual.

She said it was difficult to tell but there was a slightly higher risk in someone who had already had it than the average woman in the street: one in eight as opposed to one in nine. She then told me about her friend who had breast cancer ten years ago when she was younger than me.

I mentioned living twenty years – I would be very happy with that. She said, 'Ah, but when you've got twenty, you'll want another twenty.' Too bloody right, I will. Her friend's grandmother also had breast cancer and lived to her nineties. Bring it on!

I am more and more convinced that I should live my healthy life and, as Alison K said, I must be absolutely convinced if it did come back again that I have done what I can to stay healthy.

Osh went up to the farm today with Julia so that I could be free of him tomorrow when I have the chemo. He was hysterical when he left and I thought how traumatising it must be for Julia. Then I remembered she takes children off people for a living, so is probably used to it – plus I would actually be getting Osh back.

December 13, Wednesday

Richard and John the builders came when I was at chemo and fitted the multi-fuel burners. Hurrah, at last we will not freeze to death, although the temperature is currently about 13 degrees so I'm not sure if I will ever use them. Plus I have to assemble the bloody things inside which will take another week, no doubt, so I'm not even sure they will get lit before Christmas. I'll get Rhodri on the case next week.

Chemo day was less anxious this time although I still feel physically sick going there and even writing about it makes me feel sick. I usually have the constitution of an ox.

Thank God there are only two more treatments. I should thank my lucky stars they are so straightforward, I know.

Rachel was there again. I'm not sure exactly what she is doing, she's going to ask her supervisor for a little bit more guidance. I just rattled on about Christmas and stuff and said she could visit me at home if she liked but other than that, unless she has some questions, I don't know what her function is, nice as she is.

Felt tired and slept in the afternoon. Rhodri picked Elis up and took him to a screening of one of his programmes, so I was in the house on my own until seven and slept for a bit until Elis came home with sausage and chips. I had to nick a small bowl of chips for quality control even though I've just spent twenty minutes sending an email to Rhodri's mother on the perils of fried food! Do as I say, not as I do.

December 14, Thursday

I am very tired;, have been sleeping on and off all day. Can't really do much but definitely do not feel as bad as the last time, when I had a job to get out of bed at all because of the sickness. Acupuncture definitely works. Apart from feeling sleepy, I am very well, and to be honest it won't hurt to just do nothing for a few days. Also, it helps that I don't have Osh, much as I love him. I don't know what I would do without my wonderful mother. She looks like she needs a good holiday herself. I was wondering what I could get her for Christmas, so bought two tickets for us to go to see *Lord of the Dance* in March together.

December 15, Friday

I had a wonderful night last night, took two herbal sleeping tablets and was out for the count. What a difference it makes to how you feel, when you've had a good night's sleep. Went to Tescos this afternoon, not for anything major, spent £133, bloody hell, and that was a small shop. Granted, I had a few Christmas nibbles in there, plus stuff for Elis's party bags which cost about twenty quid. His party is on 7 February and I want to get it organised before Christmas so that I don't have to think about it then. Later, I took Elis up to the farm with Rhodri, as he is going away with Julia and Martin and Lloyd for the weekend in the Nant Ddu lodge near Brecon. Good old Julia and Martin – their reward will be in heaven. It's beautiful up there; it's near a lake and you can go walking and there's a pool for the children.

Rhodri and I went up there for a night once, it was really lovely. Actually, thinking about it, we had a big row BUT we did have a bit of nookie in a fisherman's hut the next morning, so it couldn't have been that big a row in the end.

December 16, Saturday

Ah, I have so tempted fate with the good night's sleep. Didn't sleep a bloody wink last night. I have been reading about melatonin. There is a link between it and breast cancer. Melatonin is the chemical released when you sleep, so basically the upshot of it is, you need to get lots of sleep. I am getting myself and Rhodri to bed early so our melatonin can do good things to our bodies while we sleep.

Anyway, it was about twelve o'clock and so as not to disturb Rhodri I went to the bunks, which is usually fine. But I didn't sleep. I was too hot, too cold, the bed was too small, everything was wrong and by 7.30 I was glad to get up.

The up-side of my sleeplessness was that I was like a zombie on acid and made copious amounts of red, amber and green vegetarian foods for the freezer. Now I won't have to cook much next week. After all that health-food cooking I went to Charlie Chalks with Rhodri and Osh and had scampi and chips. Osh ran about a bit, but wanted to come home so we came back and Osh fell asleep on the sofa. Rhodri and I had a half-hour sleep in bed and we had a bit of sex for old times' sake. Sex is surprisingly not at the forefront of my mind these days and I keep saying to Rhodri, 'In sickness and in health,' because I stupidly think that if I do not have sex with my husband he will leave me for another woman. Which he will not, and if he did he wouldn't have deserved such a wonderful wife and mother as me in the first place, so there.

I cleaned the goldfish out. I wonder if I stopped feeding them and cleaning their tank, whether anyone would notice (apart from Fishy and Rods, of course).

December 17, Sunday

I had an amazing dream about marriage. Yes, I know it sounds crazy but it was spiritually uplifting. I must be thinking about the things Deborah has said about being vulnerable and not talking to Rhodri about my illness and basically burying my head in the sand. I was in a really plush hotel and there was this young woman, I have no idea who she was, but she was beautiful with long blonde hair and newly married and she said that she wasn't sure if her marriage would work. She asked me what I thought marriage was and I said, as if I was a prophet or something, this:

'Marriage is about trust. Each of you must trust the other. It is about compromise and more compromise, even at times when you don't want to have to feel you have backed down or lost an argument. It is about taking a deep breath and realising that there are some things you need to stand back from. When you have been together for a long time, like my ten years with Rhodri, it is not about lamenting the passion you had at the beginning of your relationship and grieving over the loss, it is about remembering it and realising that every now and then that spark reignites, and although the intensity of those first few years is not there, it is replaced by a stronger, longer-lasting passion; that of being together and facing what life has to throw at you, holding hands tightly, as it does so. Even though there are times when you cannot stand the sight of the person you share your life with, and their voice, their touch, annoys you, it is about knowing and remembering and understanding that the balance comes when their voice and their touch alone can comfort you and make you a whole person again.'

I said to the young woman: 'You have not faced any difficulties in your life, and you will not necessarily have bad experiences, but there will be adjustments, with children or new jobs or different paths in life, and the important thing is to remember that each hurdle that you face, whatever comes your way, if you face it together you will be stronger.'

And I woke up, and it was just like the dreams you read about in the Bible, when suddenly everything in life fits into place and there is a certainty about it. I realised that all these years of thinking that my relationship with Rhodri was one hard slog, and that he can be selfish, and that he's not in touch with his emotions, and that the passion was no longer in our relationship; that this is one long steep learning curve, this is a continuum and there are really good times and not so good times but you hold on to each other through both those times.

And I thought about what we have been through, in a really short time together, in the grand scheme of things. I had a miscarriage, he was ill for six months with his back and couldn't walk and had to have an operation. We had two children, neither of whom came into the world easily, and I was ill and depressed after Elis. I've changed jobs, we've moved house and I've had cancer. We've come through an amazing amount of stuff and we are stronger for it all. We are here together and hopefully are going to grow old together for, in many, many ways, it is the shit life throws at you that makes you stronger.

I'm not going to rest on my prophetic laurels though. I will still be carting him off to the counsellor when I get over my treatment.

December 18, Monday

Ding dong, merrily on high. Still wondering about my choice of career after visiting Deborah in her lovely big house and sobbing into a hanky for an hour.

I arrived five minutes early and she said I was early, so I

had to hang around outside as if I was waiting to go into a youth club. I rang Kerry on the mobile for a time check and she said she wasn't the speaking clock – whose number I couldn't remember anyway.

So I got to the session at 10.15 EXACTLY and Deborah was trying to probe me on failing to turn up at the correct time for my last appointment. She was trying to read something deep and significant into it and despite my saying I simply lost my diary, suggested there was some subliminal reason for me not turning up.

No, I just have to write everything down and she said (I paraphrase here) that I present this calm exterior, an organised person, but there seems to be chaos around me. I said I HAVE to write everything down because I have a problem with numbers, but she kept on and on about the significance of my not turning up and suggesting that I was upset when I left – I wasn't.

I was just annoyed that I was messing her about. She went on about the diary and not being able to remember things, and that I couldn't possibly keep in my head information like an appointment, and that my sessions with her were about me and yet she thought that I saw them as unimportant.

I said that my head was so full of trivia I couldn't possibly remember everything, that's why I have the diary. I have to remember if I've given Osh some Calpol for his cold, does Elis have a handkerchief in his school bag? Does he have his money for the school trip? Are their shoes clean? Have they eaten enough fruit? Where is their vitamin C coming from? (not sure they have had any today, thinking of it, apart from in tablet form – see, there I go again). And that's all within about fifteen minutes of them being about to leave the house in the morning.

I said the diary was my way of organising the chaos and I was annoyed with myself because I only have about three appointments a week, and I can't even keep those. I felt a bit, 'Oh my God, am I the only person in the world who can't keep appointments and has to write everything down?'

My house is tidy one minute and like a tip the next and I am NEVER on top of things. I do live in a permanent chaotic state, but when you are essentially a single parent for part of the time who has been diagnosed with a life-threatening illness and for one week in three can't really do much, being too knackered with treatment, then surely keeping my bloody diary is a little link to sanity and I should be applauded for it? Except I must keep it in a safe place, otherwise the whole system collapses if I lose it.

And then along came Nigella Lawson. I saw her being interviewed on telly and they asked how she managed to keep on top of everything. She said, 'I have to make lists for everything. I need orders, and my lists tell me what to do.'

Without my lists I would be lost to the world – nothing would function in this house without my lists in THAT diary. Nigella is married to a multi-millionaire and is probably one in her own right too, she is a busy working mum AND probably has staff and she has also had tragedy in her life. And although her house is probably always tidy (apart from that room where she and Charles keep Tracy Emin's tent, or is it her bed?) even SHE has to have her lists to make order out of the chaos – thank you, thank you, thank you, Nigella. I will refer Deborah to Nigella if she EVER asks me about my bloody diary again.

The session with Deborah (apart from Diarygate) was very good and I was going on ad infinitum about my marriage, saying I had shared some of my shit with Rhodri and that it hadn't made me feel that great because I was unburdening on him. But that he sent me some roses and I realised that sharing the burden is good.

I told her that I had asked him about my illness and that it occurred to me that I had not asked him in six months what he thought about my cancer, and what he had said. 'I'm not sure what all this has to do with my cancer,' I remarked, 'I seem to be fixated on my marriage.'

She said that Rhodri was the person I was turning to in my time of need, and as he physically wasn't there at a time when I needed him, perhaps I was thinking I needed him because I can't do this on my own. She's right (of course she is bloody right, she's a highly paid counsellor).

She asked me who I talked to about my illness in any detail and I said no one, and that's it, I don't. I am the jolly cancer victim protecting those around me because I don't want them to be hurt by my pain. That is hard work and it is impossible to keep going and sometimes you have to break down and cry and I have thought that crying would be letting the cancer get the better of me, but it is also a way of dealing with the cancer. You HAVE to tell someone all those thoughts and fears that are on your mind, because I think if you don't confront those demons, no matter how frightening they may be, they will catch up with you at some point. Better out than in.

She asked me what I had thought about coming to see her and I told her that I had been sceptical about it, that I had thought no one could understand me better than me, that I had analysed myself in depth and thought there was nothing else to know.

I said that I had found that wasn't the case, and that she had opened my eyes to a lot of things about myself that I had never thought of, that I am vulnerable but the way I deal with that is putting up this front which no one can penetrate and I was learning to show my emotions to Rhodri, because if he didn't know about them he can't begin to understand them.

I said I was a 'horrible' perfectionist and she asked me why I used the word 'horrible' and I said, 'Because being this perfectionist all the time is hard work, actually it's exhausting.' Always thinking that everything has to be just right takes up time and energy, and having to be the best at everything and never failing at anything and expecting everyone around me, especially Rhodri, to live up to those standards drains all your energy. I have lived my life trying to be perfect at everything.

Then I said, 'The thing is, I've realised that I'm not perfect. I have flaws, some quite fundamental ones, and for years I have thought that Rhodri was the one who was unreasonable and emotionally closed when actually I think it was me who was those things.'

She said I presented this image to the world of being in control and calm. I said, yes, but it was like stage management, because inside I am a mess sometimes, and situations and people in authority make me nervous, but I keep this front up and it's bloody hard work.

She said that my body wasn't perfect, that I had cancer, and I said that I thought that realisation was making me look at my life in a different way. My name is Michelle and I am not perfect and I am so bloody relieved that I never have to be perfect again.

December 19, Tuesday

Ding dong merrily on high . . . Hosanna in excelsis, la la la la la la la la . . . Kerry came over with baby Daisy today and we wrapped all the presents in the attic, which were threatening to come through the ceiling. There were hundreds of them. It took the two of us nearly four hours (interspersed with tea breaks and lunch).

We were listening to all the old favourites: Bing Crosby and all those other old crooners singing Christmas songs, I had my log-burner going and it was all lovely and Christmassy.

Later, when the children had gone to bed, because the back room was so nice with the wood-burner, Rhodri and I stayed out there and Rhodri went out to get a pizza and a bottle of cava (didn't sit well with my no wheat, no cheese, no alcohol – but for God's sake you are a long time dead) and we did the After Dinner Quiz – well in our case the During Dinner quiz. He was so pissed off because I was ahead all the time, in truth he thinks that I know nothing, and when I said the grey squirrel was introduced from North America, he said he wasn't going to give it to me as there was no such country as North America. Oh, how I love beating him in quizzes.

I said, 'You hate it because you don't think I know anything.' The truth is, although the questions can be difficult, there is some logic to them. Example: *Who is the Patron Saint of Carpenters?* Just think of the most famous carpenter – Joseph – and there's your answer. He thinks I am some mad genius for being able to retain this info when I'm just guessing and he (being a man) does not realise that my brain simply does not have enough room to retain the Patron Saint of Carpenters, even if I wanted to. But like every other bit of thinking I do on my feet there's some logic somewhere, it's just a question of finding it.

December 20, Wednesday

George Clooney is the single most handsome man on this planet and I defy ANY woman to say otherwise. He is handsome and clever and knows where Darfur is and all those terrible things that are going on there (I am Googling it as I write) and can act and direct and never kisses and tells.

Anyway, I dreamt that I was actually going out with him last night – that we were an item – and it was so real, and I was ringing Kerry up talking about George and Brad Pitt, who are good friends, and I said – in my dream, on the phone to Kerry, 'Listen to me talking about George and

160

Brad' – and then I woke up.

BUT I'm sure I would have something meaningful to say to George, if I ever met him, especially now I have Googled Darfur. Fucking hell, it's grim out there. There are 450,000 people dead and 2.5 million displaced. It's a country run by genocidal maniacs and I know bugger all about it. It has taken a dream about George Clooney to educate me. Thank you, George. I will donate some of my Christmas money to the cause.

Went to see Ian J today. Will that man ever get a bloody wife and be as miserable as the rest of us? I told him that Elis asked out of the blue the other day, 'Why doesn't Ian have a wife?' I said that he was trying very hard, but I really don't think he is.

He's there with his bloody cats and his bachelor existence in a house where, if you put something away, it stays put away. He has a garden that is perfect and he can pop to the shops anytime he wants: and can use a whole trolley without any small bodies riding inside it.

And he can go to football and to a pub, and is answerable to no one except, ultimately, God. He needs to suffer like the rest of us.

Did the quiz again with Rhodri and he beat me by one point. Unlike him, I am gracious in defeat.

December 21, Thursday

Joanne and my mother came down today and did a pre-Christmas clean for me. I protested and said I would rather they just came to visit me, but they insisted and I was very glad by the end of it as it would have taken me all day. But with three of us it was a few hours and it does look so lovely when it is clean and tidy. My IKEA open-plan living dream is there in all its minimalist glory for all of one hour before I had to pick the children up.

I am resolving to put everything away and keep it clean before Sioned and Ali come on Saturday for Christmas.

Babs came round and we ate mince pies. I have eaten four of them today and I don't even like the things. Now I'm scared to get on the scales as I can feel I have put on weight. Oh well. I will diet after chemo. I need all my mince-pie strength to face my treatment.

December 22, Friday

I dropped Elis and Osh off in school and nursery and on the way Elis was singing 'Here it is, Merry Christmas, everybody's having fun,' and I saw two builders looking over and I smiled at them, thinking they were thinking my little Christmas angel was cute.

Walked back to the house after I dropped the kids off at school and nursery and I heard one builder say to the other, 'It's her,' and he came out from behind a wall and smiled and I smiled back and he was quite nice and buildery and then I walked on and they wolf-whistled – TWICE. I could not believe it: TWO BUILDERS FANCIED ME.

I forgot that I was once a radical feminist who would have turned around and stuck her fingers up at them, I just walked on with my head held high, beaming. I wanted to whip my wig off and say, 'Aha!, I have no hair and cancer and someone still fancies me who isn't my husband.'

Alison K was in the house with Erin and Rhodri when I got back.. I was like an excited schoolgirl. I said, 'Alison, I know you won't approve but two builders just whistled at me and it was bloody great.'

Spent the day with Alison K and Erin mooching about IKEA. Alison K went for some plates for her Christmas nutloaf and I just went along for the ride really, having done all my Christmas things and not having to cook a bloody thing (hurrah!) as Ali is doing us an Iranian meal for Christmas dinner and he is the most wonderful cook ever.

We shopped around, then had lunch, then Erin played and we had coffee and then it was school picking-up time. We spent the entire afternoon discussing mad families at Christmas – hers and mine. I would tell a story, then she would say, 'Well, listen to this . . . ' Then we discussed people who have or want affairs (not us, though) and decided that they really had to 'get over it' where children were concerned.

I do of course realise that life is not always as simple as that, and I never thought I would actually say this, but I highly value the sanctity of marriage and bringing children up within it. If Rhodri leaves me, EVER, now I value the sanctity of marriage, I will never forgive him.

It is the last day of school today and I had promised Elis he could have two of his schoolfriends over. He has been counting the days down all week – four sleeps to Jonah and Ben coming over, three sleeps to Jonah and Ben coming over, etcetera. Anyway, he has been as excited about them coming as he has about Christmas. So I opened the curtains and I said what Elis always says when the day he has been counting sleeps to finally arrives, 'Tomorrow's today!' And he jumped up, and Rhodri, who had been sleeping in the Bob the Builder bunk, jokingly said, 'Yeah, Merry Christmas,' and I jokingly said, 'Yeah, let's see if he's been,' and with that Elis ran downstairs thinking it was Christmas morning. Then I said, 'Oh no, it's not Christmas really, it's Ben and Jonah day, that's what I meant,' and he said slightly dejectedly, 'Oh, I thought it was Christmas.'

I always think it is a good idea, especially as it makes Elis the happiest boy on the planet, to have two of his friends over but then I remember that two energetic boys are enough; four is too many. My mother had four children, albeit four girls, and when I went on holiday with Kate in the summer and we had four children to look after between the two of us, I was exhausted when I got back, and said to my mother, 'How on earth did you keep going with four all the time?'

She said, 'I never took you anywhere.' Fair point, if you don't go anywhere, you can't get stressed. She is right, we never did go anywhere but were basically left to run wild around woods and hills, with her not knowing from one hour to the next where we were. Can you imagine that happening now? If they are out of your sight for five minutes you think a homicidal paedophile has kidnapped your kids. It certainly was a different time.

Anyway I stopped outside the nursery with the three boys in the back talking about poo and nappies and Osh, and I jokingly said, 'Well, it wasn't that long ago you three were in nappies,' to which they all recoiled in horror. I continued, 'I remember changing Elis's nappy.' Ben and Jonah taunted him and he was crying in the car, so we all had to say sorry to Elis to stop him crying and I had to deny that I could ever remember changing his nappy, oh no, I was only joking and it was all all right then.

I warned them that if they moved out of the car while I went in to pick Osh up, Father Christmas would not be coming to them. When I went in to get Osh, he had soiled his nappy so I asked if the staff would mind changing him as I had to keep an eye on the three boys through the window. I turned round to check on them and all three blond-haired, blue-eyed, six-year-old angels were out of the car on the elevated grass bank opposite the BBC (where I work and am respected) and they all had their todgers out, pissing in the air and swaying back and forth showing them to the traffic below, cheering like drunken football fans after an away win. I went out and said in my primmest voice, 'Back in the car – immediately!' Obviously the Father Christmas threat didn't work and I wondered how I was going to control them all for the next few hours.

I took them all to McDonald's (cop out I know, but at least they will eat it) and they were rather loud and noisy, but boys will be boys and it's just nice to see them so happy. Then they played in the house for a few hours and Rhodri took them home. Ah, peace and quiet. If I could have stayed at home and had children earlier, and found out how much I enjoyed being a mother, I would have had more children, but life doesn't work like that. I have two healthy, happy little boys and am grateful to God, or whatever greater good is out there that gave me them, every day.

December 23, Saturday

Sioned and Ali are arriving later and, big excitement, we are going to Waitrose en famille. Waitrose surely is *the* Christmas supermarket. We never go shopping together en famille because 1) Rhodri is never around to go shopping and 2) it is much too stressful. However, when there are two adults and two children and Osh can have an entire trolley to himself without a single item annoying him, then it is luxury.

There is a depressing air about Waitrose. It's an upmarket supermarket, to serve the very posh Vale of Glamorgan, but located in the downmarket town of Barry, which is surrounded by a chemical works. You could never sell your house if you lived there, except to someone else who worked in the chemical works. It is like something out of *Blade Runner* – I kid you not.

You have all these posh people in their 4 x 4's putting truffles in their trolleys, and outside you have people who can't afford to come in the door. All of this made me feel slightly uncomfortable. Maybe they can put some trees around the houses by the chemical works so the eyes of the middle-classes are not offended.

It was really quiet in Waitrose, with lovely food, although, lots of it had sold out, and reassuringly expensive (won't be going again). I remembered also when I went there why I haven't been supermarket shopping with Rhodri for years, because he undermines my purchasing. I put something in the trolley and he gets it out again and we end up having an argument about the merits of the said item in the middle of the supermarket.

Osh was in his element with a trolley (train as he calls it) all to himself and he sat in it being very cute, shouting at the top of his voice, 'Merry Christmas, everybody!' over and over again.

Sioned and Ali arrived with enough food for two Christmases and they looked after the children while Rhodri and I went out for a meal with Alison K, Neil and Ian J and his friend Helen to the local Indian, where we all ate, drank and were Christmas merry.

December 24, Sunday

Christmas Eve is here at last. The sweets in the Advent calendars are all present and correct: there is one left in each. Elis has finally acknowledged that Santa is coming tomorrow; he has been saying for some time it is today and has called me a 'liar', a word I do not like at all, because I was saying it is tomorrow, which it was not. I now have to host Owain and Eva, Rhodri's brother and shiny new wife, and Rhodri's parents for lunch. No one got out of bed until eleven – well, I say no one, I was up about seven with two children but the others were nowhere to be seen. However, when they got up they sprang into action and within a short space of time there was a lovely feast on the table fit for a king. We all tucked into lunch and exchanged gifts to be opened on Christmas day.

I had a little sleep in the afternoon – well, tried to, as it was slightly chaotic with the children. We had a sort of shift system, with girls first (me and Sioned) then boys (Rhodri and Ali) so we all got a rest.

My father came down with Elis's bike (his present from my parents) and stayed for a bit talking to Sioned and Ali.

I managed to get the children to bed early after doing the reindeer food: a carrot, a mince pie, a glass of wine, and establishing where Santa was going to put the presents. I lay in bed with the two little bodies reading *Away in a Manger* (the story of the nativity) and *'Twas the Night Before Christmas* – I love that poem – to get them all Christmased up for tomorrow. Osh went off to sleep and Elis and I lay in bed chatting about Santa and what he might bring. Martyn rang when I was in bed. I had my phone in my pocket and I was chatting to him and wished him Merry Christmas. When I put the phone down, Elis thought that I had been talking to Santa. I had to wait some time then to make sure Elis was fast asleep – I couldn't face the thought of ruining the Christmas myth for him.

So then we put all the presents out, which took some time, and there was a ridiculous amount of stuff. Every year I say I'm not going to buy much and every year I do.

Anyway, I then remembered the bike in the shed (thankfully) and Rhodri had to get it out and Ali and Sioned spent about half an hour wrapping it meticulously. We drank some wine and we went to bed.

December 25, Monday

Christmas-time. Mistletoe and rhyme . . . It's here at last, Christmas Day. Rhodri and I are sleeping in Elis's room as Sioned and Ali have our room. There are two mattresses on the floor; they were supposed to be for me and Rhodri to sleep on as a couple but Rhodri said it would spark his allergy to dust off so Elis and I are on the mattresses on the floor and Rhodri is in the bunk (very romantic).

I had been awake for about half an hour (it was about seven thirty) just waiting for Elis to wake up – not a peep from Osh next door – thinking I couldn't go down for a cup of tea as Elis might wake up and come down and it might spoil the spirit of Christmas. So I was waiting and he got up and went to the toilet and came back. I said to him, 'Do you remember what day it is?' and he said, 'Yes, it's Christmas.' I said, 'Shall we go down and see if Santa has left you anything?' and he said, 'No, thanks, I feel a bit sick.' So I lay next to him feeling his forehead for a minute, thinking he might really be ill but he seemed OK, then he said, 'OK, let's go down now.' I think the anticipation was all too much for him.

Of course we then had to get Osh up and Rhodri up and Sioned and Ali up before Elis could go down, and by this time he was like a racehorse at the starting gate. Finally, all assembled, all present and correct at the landing roll call, we went downstairs and, 'He's been!' and it was a mad frenzy. Osh didn't know what had hit him; Elis was just ripping at things like a semi-madman. Osh meticulously opened a present then had to have it out of the box immediately before going on to the next present (which meant he was all morning opening his stuff until Elis helped out). It was a really lovely morning, all captured on video and film, of course.

The house looks as if someone has ransacked it. Christmas lunch was amazing; we had chicken and coriander with aubergine and tomato and rice and salad and mint dips and champagne. It was mmm. As my mother always says at the end of a Christmas Day, 'It's as far away now as it will ever be.'

December 26, Tuesday

Boxing Day is Cardiff City Day in our house: a family tradition stretching back to when Elis was born and, coincidentally, Rhodri embraced Cardiff City with a vengeance. Elis was born and within a few short months Rhodri had become this fanatical Cardiff City fan and buggered off every other weekend to watch the match. It used to be a big bone of contention between us as we'd both be working all week then come Saturday he'd be out all day and I'd be left literally holding the baby. I guess I've just got used to it now but if he EVER EVER suggested away games I'd be cutting up his Ambassadors membership for sure.

I don't go as I have never understood all the fuss about football, but Elis and Rhodri went with Jonah and Peter his dad. Elis has become as fanatical as Rhodri about football; talk about in your own image. He comes down of a morning now and instead of putting on his usual cartoons, he checks out the league tables. He's six, for God's sake. I didn't even know what they were until I was about twenty. He will also watch obscure leagues on Sky Sports like the German League and he comes in to ask Rhodri which side he should be supporting.

Sioned and Ali and Osh and I went for a walk around Roath Park. We walked all around the park and our treat was to be a coffee when we got around, but as we arrived at the café it was shutting! It was very cold out, freezing in fact, so we went home to coffee and chocolate cake to try to warm ourselves up a bit.

We did our girl/boy sleeping rota again and I slept for about two hours. So far we have eaten, drunk and slept our way through Christmas.

December 27, Wednesday

Went to Branwen and Patrick's house today with Rhodri, Elis, Osh and Sioned and Ali, or Ali and Ali, as Osh is calling them for some reason. Ali is Ali and Sioned is 'and Ali' or sometimes just Ali, so Osh is following her around the house going, 'Come on, Ali.' He will NOT have it that her name is Sioned. It is very funny.

Rhodri's parents were there, we had coffee and I sat at the kitchen table and made things out of Play Doh, as you do. Then we went up to my mother's house and she made us all turkey and chips, which I ate with a huge amount of white bread and pickled onions. Christmas is perfect now. Sioned and Ali went back to London so Rhodri and I, or should I say me barking orders at Rhodri, took the opportunity to tidy up and get a bit of order back in our house which is bursting at the seams with stuff and will have even more stuff when it is Elis's party so I have to find homes for this stuff to make way for the other stuff that will follow. Lloyd is coming for a sleepover tonight.

December 28, Thursday

Lloyd went to bed quite early last night. He was exhausted, a bit Christmased out and had a little cry for his mummy, but it didn't last long. I think he just needed to sleep. Elis came down and watched a bit of telly with us. Lloyd and Elis are only two years apart but Elis is not really into fantasy role playing until Lloyd comes down, so they spent all last night and today being Jedi Knights and Power Rangers, both united against one evil – Osh.

Osh is their mortal enemy, which means running away from him and screaming at the top of their voices every time he comes near them. Instead of being phased by all of this, Osh runs after them screaming and making monster noises at them. Lloyd is obsessed with Osian touching anything that belongs to him – he thinks he will break it. He is also a great teller of tales which is very handy because if Osh does the slightest naughty thing, he will come down and tell me.

Osh is such a good sport for a small wee thing and had, I thought, no idea he was actually their mortal enemy and the aim was to keep him out of the bedroom. He is slightly more canny than I thought, though, as I heard him saying to Lloyd rather wearily, 'Don't kill me any more, Lloyd. Can you stop killing me now?' So I intervened and made them all play 'nicely' together which is all any mummy with three screaming juvenile Christmas maniacs round her wants to do. Julia and Martin came to pick him up suitably hungover – they had stayed the night in a hotel in Cardiff with their friends. I was for once in my life quietly smug that Julia has a hangover, as I have spent my life being in the shadow of her control and self-restraint where alcohol is concerned.

December 29, Friday

Rhodri has gone to work. He was making this big point of keeping Osh off nursery like some Victorian dad with his, 'No child of mine goes to nursery over Christmas,' then informs me THIS MORNING that he is going to work today. I was bloody furious and had Osh in the crèche within fifteen minutes of this announcement, kicking and screaming as I left him, wailing, 'Mummy , Mummy!' I have to admit, much as I love my little angel, I didn't look back and had a bit of a skip in my step knowing I didn't have the 24/7 responsibility for him. They always stop crying the minute you leave them anyway – at least, that's what they tell you in the nursery.

Elis and I went to Techniquest as part of my great

Christmas Plan to spend one-to-one quality time with him. Osh gets me to himself a lot of the time as Rhodri tends to do things with Elis more. I was on the way to Techniquest when a fire engine passed us and I said, 'Oh, I hope that's not going to Techniquest,' and when we got there it was. They had evacuated the place so we went for lunch; I tried to persuade Elis that hummus and olives in the Millennium Centre were preferable to an American-style diner but unfortunately that argument falls on deaf ears with a six year old, so we went to the American-style diner which he thought was great, of course, and insisted on sitting next to me like you would on a 'date'.

He has a mild interest in going on a date but at this stage of his life it is only with me (first option) or with Rhodri (second option). I apparently would have to pay as he doesn't have any money, which is exactly what happened the first time his father and I went on a date. A chip off the old block, no doubt.

At the moment though, he is very anti-girls and says 'Yuck!' every time anything remotely girly comes on TV – a habit which Osh has now picked up on. He wants to live with either Ben or Jonah, his two friends from school, depending on where his allegiances lie at the time. This needs to happen apparently so that they can live in a flat, drink beer and watch football with no babies around them, and even when they are old 'mans', as Elis puts it, they will still be watching football, so there you have it – Elis's life-plan.

Techniquest had reopened by the time we finished lunch and we went in. My period started on Christmas Day and has got progressively worse ever since. It is not at all painful but is very heavy and I have been getting clots. But this has been nothing, no, nothing, compared to what I experienced in Techniquest. It was basically like someone had turned on a tap. Like having a miscarriage without the pain. There were enormous blood clots and lots of blood. I kept having to go to the toilet. I didn't like leaving Elis in the play area on his own so I kept dragging him along with me to the toilet. After the third time I did this I had to let him just play on his own, on pain of death he wouldn't move out of the building, and if ANYONE approached him he was to start screaming and kick them and say, 'I don't know you!' at the top of his voice. I hope that never backfires and he doesn't use it on me, getting me carted off to the local police station.

Anyway, I had to change my towel about six times in an hour and a half. In the end I just sat on the toilet for about ten minutes as there was no point leaving it. It was a bloody nightmare. It stopped eventually but it left me feeling really drained.

Got home and looked up chemo and periods on the internet. This is a very common side effect, apparently (thanks for telling me, everyone). I thought I was going to have my periods obliterated and live a life free of the evil curse, but no, instead they come with a vengeance.

December 30, Saturday

Kerry, Richard C, Daisy and Felix are coming tomorrow to stay for New Year's Eve and Ian J is coming along too, but not staying. Ah, the old gang reunited under one roof with the addition of four children aged three months to six, nearly seven, years. So Rhodri and I tided the house to within an inch of its life and it looked like something out of a magazine for all of one afternoon. I guess this is how your house looks if you have 'help' or 'servants' as Elis likes to call anyone who waits on you.

Rhodri, Elis and my father went to the football, Osh watched the telly and I made a Beef Bourguignon for tomorrow so I wouldn't have to be cooking all day. I bought a nut roast for Ian J which is a huge cop out, but serves him right for being a vegetarian.

December 31, Sunday

Nearly the end of another year, a rather eventful one in the Williams-Huw household – well, for me certainly. The children wouldn't have noticed, although they will of course benefit for years to come from the new enlightened me. Felix and Osh played really well together and we all had a really nice time. Kerry and I were just itching to get the champagne started (we had four bottles in total) but didn't dare touch a drop until all the children were tucked up in their beds.

Ian J came round and I told Rhodri everything was prepared, he just had to cook the potatoes and heat it all up as I was too tipsy to possibly co-ordinate anything and, hey presto, a gourmet New Year's Eve dinner. We got on the champagne with a vengeance and were quite pissed within about an hour. The food was a triumph – thanks, Delia, for the recipe and to me for being, when I want to be, a fabulous cook. Everyone wanted seconds, even Ian with his nut roast (a triumph for Tesco, no doubt).

Osh woke up about 11.30 p.m. and came downstairs by himself and was watching Scooby Doo in the other room.

New Year started with a bang from the fireworks outside and hugs and kisses all round, including a few group hugs (we were very pissed by this time), and Osh was here to celebrate it with us. The others slept soundly through it all.

I sat at the kitchen table and for a little while just looked at the others in the adjoining room – Richard lying out on the sofa, Kerry sitting beside him, Ian and Rhodri with their playful banter. I felt a bit like the happy-go-lucky me, before I had cancer, with a glass of champagne in my hand and the company of my dearest friends, laughing and joking like I didn't have a care in the world.

January 1, Monday

Another New Year. I have no resolutions as the biggest vice I have is coffee and I am not giving that up, PLUS I have spent the last six months resolving to change just about everything there could possibly be, so figure this is one year I will give up giving up.

Rhodri made us go for a New Year's walk by the sea; to say it was bracing is a mild understatement. We went in those beautiful walled gardens by the sea in Southern Down, which lead up to the top of the cliff, and the sea was just in turmoil, crashing against the cliffs. It was howling a gale by the time we reached the top of the cliff, which meant we came back down with the full force of the wind and the rain, and Osh was so cold and so wet, he kept crying so much, that Elis and I had to try hard not to laugh as he felt so sorry for himself.

Needless to say I was horribly hungover and did not mind too much having the rain lashing against my face; it was almost comforting. My wig was hilarious. When I got back in the car, I looked like one of those people in a sketch show where it is so obvious they are wearing a wig. Unlike real hair, when they are blown about by the wind, wings tend to stay in that position, rather than flopping back down when the wind has subsided. All I needed was a chin strap and the sketch-show look would have been complete. Needed to have curry and chips though, when we got back as a hangover cure.

January 2, Tuesday

It's seven years to the day my little beautiful boy Elis was born. A millennium baby. He was actually due on Christmas Eve but decided to pop out on 2 January. Well, not exactly pop out – it was a rather long protracted affair and despite myself, every time I drive past the hospital where he was born I get a little reminder of the horror that is childbirth.

But you do forget; I went on to have Osh, and his birth was even more horrendous. I ended up giving birth to him on my own as the nurse went to get me a paracetamol. I had said to her, 'I think I'm in labour, I know what being in labour is like,' and she said, 'No, you couldn't possibly be. I'll get you a paracetamol.'

I said, 'I think I'm going to need something stronger than a paracetamol.' But she ignored me and left, and I gave birth to Osh in bed on my own. The only thing that stopped him falling on the floor was that he got caught in my knickers – something to thank Tesco for, the durability of their knickers. Elis's birth was about twelve hours, not so bad but I lost so much blood after it that I couldn't get out of bed for about ten days.

That's a bit what having the chemo is like, only a milder version; it sort of wipes you out, like after you've had a baby and you feel the sleep deprivation that you can only get in that situation.

I went to the hospital for a blood test and shamelessly cheated the queue, telling Gill it was my little boy's birthday and I had promised to take him to Toys R Us. Who could possibly refuse a cancer patient that?

When I told Gill about my periods, she said it was normal. I said my red bloods might be affected because it was pretty bad, I had lost a lot of blood and felt a bit washed-out. She told me about another of her patients who actually couldn't go out, it was so bad. Bloody hell, there is always someone who is worse than you, isn't there?

She said the periods might get even heavier or they might stop. I thought that if you had them throughout your chemo they would carry on. If they continue being as bad as they have been, I will seriously have to do something about them, like my sister who had the ovarian ablation, as I just could not live with them. I couldn't sit in a meeting or go on a car journey like that, it would be impossible. I have four months now essentially without the chemo and before I go back to work, so I will see how they go.

I also need to fully discuss my options with the Tamoxifen and having my ovaries removed. Although I have to say the thought of having more surgery, especially surgery which knocks you out for a few weeks, as opposed to a few days with my breast surgery, is not appealing as I am coming to the end of my treatment.

It may be that when I've finished Tamoxifen – the drug that stops oestrogen from getting to the breast and feeding the cancer – I will want to have them removed. BUT if my periods continue like this, then I cannot live with it; I might as well have my ovaries removed as have an ovarian ablation. I can't believe I have to think about these things.

Although my mother told me that she had her ovaries removed when she was forty-two – she had an eptopic pregnancy, so she also had an early menopause – she was on those bloody HRT plasters for years. I couldn't go on them, I probably cannot take anything to address my menopause if I have one, but I know that diet and exercise and running into the garden in the snow naked – as my mother once did – can help a lot with these hot flushes.

I figure I have to go through it sometime so it doesn't matter if I am forty or fifty – does it? I've no bloody idea what I am talking about. I need to discuss this in detail with a medical professional, methinks.

Gill rang me as I got home to say my white blood count was borderline but it was fine to have the chemo, and that my red cells were down but not enough to do anything about them yet; however, they had dipped.

I could feel they were not right though, so it was not a huge surprise.

I dropped Osh off at nursery before I went to the hospital, so we could take Elis to Toys R Us with Lloyd.

Last time we took Osh he wouldn't sit in a trolley – can you blame him when faced with thousands of toys? – and he ended up knocking about two hundred Playstation games off a shelf by putting his hand on the shelf and running to the end of the row, whereupon they all just fell on the floor. I decided I could actually live without that degree of stress on Elis's birthday this year.

Going to Toys R Us has been Elis's wish for two years in a row, after he found out there was a shop as big as a supermarket which only sold toys. He couldn't believe such a place existed until he went there – it was like taking him to Lapland. So he likes to go there and know that he can choose anything he wants from the entire store; in practice that is not true, but I know the things he wants will be within a certain price range so he lives with the illusion that he can actually have anything.

It is also his great wish that I win the lottery, then he can buy all of the toys in Toys R Us. It is also my great wish to win the lottery and have a great big house in the Vale of Glamorgan with a great big swimming pool and to shut my door and never leave the house again. But realistically I don't think it will happen, so I will be grateful for my little Llandaff semi-detached, as semi was something that I aspired to and now here I am all suburbiaed up and I didn't even have to win the lottery, just pay an enormous mortgage for the next seventeen years and never go out because I can't afford to.

I hadn't realised that Lloyd had never been to Toys R Us before, probably for the same reason we kept Osh away from the place. He kept running around looking at things and saying at the top of his voice, 'Bloody hell.' Martin, his father, says that after a day with me, Lloyd's language is terrible. True, I do say, 'Bloody hell' a lot BUT I had not uttered a single swearword up until that point, but Martin still thinks I am a bad influence, no doubt. We went to Charlie Chalks for lunch – we will not hear a bad word said against Charlie Chalks, and even though Rhodri considers himself to be something of a connoisseur of fine food, he embraces the place just as I do.

Charlie Chalks means we are able to sit down and eat a meal together while the children, after having had a mouthful of sausage, peas and chips, bugger off and play in the ball pool, leaving us in peace and not having to worry about them annoying other diners, or making too much noise as ALL of the children are like that and NO ONE gives you those looks you get in restaurants, especially from people who don't have children. They just don't understand what it is like to have to keep the kids quiet for an hour.

After a leisurely lunch, we picked Osh up from nursery, then took Elis up to the farm with Lloyd as Elis will be staying there until Sunday, when he will come back for his party in the leisure centre. Rhodri is able to take Osh to the crèche and pick him up so I don't have to worry about the children if I am not feeling well after my chemo tomorrow.

January 6, Saturday

I have lost four days of my life. Well, not exactly lost them, they were still there but they passed in a sort of drug-induced haze. I have never taken Class A drugs, but can only imagine that this is what it feels like. I have not been able to get out of bed, except yesterday I was able to come down and lie on the sofa, but even then I couldn't keep my eyes open for very long. Lack of sleep is the least of my worries this time round. Being able to stay awake for more than an hour was the problem.

It was almost instant. After the session, I came home and all I wanted to do was sleep; I was physically incapable of looking after the children or in fact doing anything. I managed to come downstairs and make myself porridge or soup and go back to bed again.

My sisters would have come down but I really wanted to be left alone to lie in my pit. I didn't want to talk to anyone. I was unable to have acupuncture the week before, because Rosie and her friend were not around, and the only other time I have felt remotely like this was when I didn't have acupuncture the week before my treatment. I know that the chemotherapy has a cumulative effect. I saw Sandra in the hospital on Tuesday – she was in when I had my op – and she said that after her fifth chemotherapy session she threw up in a supermarket.

I didn't feel particularly sick, in fact less so than previously. I have discovered that if you take Gaviscon or Milk of Magnesia, which I was knocking back, that it really offsets the nausea feeling. I stopped taking all medication after three days as opposed to five with no ill effects – I also thought maybe it was the medication that knocked me out and I did feel a lot better after stopping taking it, but that could have just been a coincidence.

I also had VERY negative feelings when I went for treatment this time. I hate the smell of the place, and as lovely as the nurses are there, I cannot stand seeing them. It's horrible, I know, because they are so chatty and are so kind, but I have no wish to see them and exchange pleasantries with them. I just want to say, 'Get me out of here.' The needle in my hand was so painful, I was crying, and then I felt ashamed because I was acting like a big baby.

Thank God Rhodri came. I was going to go on my own. Julia rang and said she would come, but I think if anyone comes with me other than Rhodri, I will be stressed. I would feel that I had to put on a brave face for them. Rhodri said late last night, almost as a throwaway comment, 'Do you want me to come?' and I said, 'Yes, please. I don't want to go on my own.' He thought that Rachel was coming but she is still away. Rachel is also good, she makes me put on a brave face too. So no Rachel, no brave face, a needle that was bloody excruciating and the smell which makes me feel like throwing up, all contributed to a very negative feeling about going to the cancer hospital – surprise surprise.

I feel sick just writing about the place – and as time has gone on it has got worse, not better. You would think it would be the reverse as I am getting to the end, but the truth is, with each visit and each session I have come to dread going to the place more and more, and no matter how much I try to pretend basically I do not want to be a cancer patient in a cancer hospital getting treatment for cancer. I want my life back, thank you very much.

I want to go to work and have people bother me with their problems to sort out, I want nothing more than to worry whether I have enough time in the lunch-hour to nip to the supermarket and then nip home to put the food in the fridge. I want to have nothing more to worry about than do I have soup for lunch or go for fish and chips in the canteen? Should I do the ironing tonight or leave it until tomorrow? Should I go out on a Wednesday for a meal with Babs or a Friday? I want my life to be filled with trivia once more. I am fed up of living my life around hospital appointments and test results and internet searches on things you never really wanted to have to think about at my age, like osteoporosis, and having your ovaries whipped out, or secondary cancer.

I have been crying on the phone to my mother as I have been very down. Alison K rang and I was really down for once with her, as I always try to be so upbeat about it all and it's just too hard to keep doing that because this time I do feel sorry for myself. I feel sorry that I have cancer at thirty-nine and that I have had to go through this and, yes, I do feel grateful that I will in all probability be cured of this cancer and I thank God every day for that and for letting me look at life with fresh eyes, but there IS a sadness also in

181

losing a bit of my life and this happening, and the truth is, the real truth, is I'd rather it wasn't happening to me.

January 7, Sunday

It was Elis's party today. We had it in the leisure centre with football on one court, a Bouncy Castle and a face painter and about thirty children. A great time was had by all. The boys were manic, they could hardly sit down to eat their food and ate their jellies before eating any other food. The girls were calm, sat down for about half an hour, ate all their food and then went on to their jellies. There is a moral or something in that somewhere.

Because I have been so unwell, wonderful, marvellous Joanne and Russell did all the party food at their house and brought it down with them. I didn't have to do a thing except turn up. I said I would make sure that next time I invited thirty children for a party, I would be ill again.

Elis and Rhodri went off after the party to see Cardiff play Spurs with Alison K, Jay and Alison's dad. As Elis got in the car and I was saying goodbye, he turned to Jay and said, 'My mummy wears a wig – does yours?' Jay did not know what a wig was, apparently.

Rhodri had arranged for Elis's photo to be put up on the big screen at the game for his birthday, and for them to say Happy Birthday over the Tannoy and they put it up about three times. It was the perfect end to his perfect day.

Osh came back with Elis for the party. I haven't seen him for a few days. He woke at eleven in the night and I went to him and he was crying, so I brought him downstairs and gave him some Calpol because he has a bad cold. Then I said I was going to bed myself. I thought he would want to go back in his own bed because he has never slept with me. Unlike Elis who was a leech on my back for years, Osh has never been the slightest bit interested in coming into bed with me, not even for a lie-in in the mornings, whereas Elis would happily stay there all day.

It was really strange because Osh got into bed and he lay down and he held my hand and looked into my eyes for ages and it was as if he was saying, 'It's OK to be ill, Mummy, we're all ill sometimes,and I'm here to look after you,' and my heart ached, it was so lovely.

January 8, Monday

Back to school today. Hurrah for a bit of normality and, to be honest, a bit of a rest. We are having new shelves and an outer front door fitted. Nigel is coming to do them, and to say the house is a bit chaotic today is an understatement. We have hundreds of books which have been in the attic for two and a half years waiting for shelves to be put up, but with all the other work we've had done on the house the shelves have rather taken a back seat.

It sort of begs the question that if we haven't seen the books for two and a half years and have had no reason to find them for reference (apart from the odd cookery book or French phrase book), do we really need them cluttering up our middle room? The answer has to be yes, ONLY because I think it is vitally important for children to grow up around books and think it is normal and natural to pluck a book off a shelf and read it.

I grew up in a house that didn't have any books. I cannot really believe it now, but we never had a bookcase. My grandmother had a bookcase at the top of her stairs and I probably read every single book in it as they were the only books I had any easy access to, apart from the Secret Seven and Famous Five series by Enid Blyton.

My grandmother also liked reading Mills & Boons; this meant I ended up reading hundreds of the bloody things and in retrospect probably explains why I have such an unrealistic view of how relationships should be, having spent most of my formative years reading about passionate love affairs ending up in happily-ever-after land.

Anyway, I left Nigel to the shelves and went off to see Deborah. For once I really felt like I needed to have my brain ironed out by her. I find I cry less in her sessions but I still get very emotional. I told her I had been ill and had been feeling sorry for myself, and was at a point where I just really wanted my life back and to get back to work and some normality.

She said (in so many words) that I am hard on myself. I say I feel bad because there are people in that hospital who are so ill they have to be brought to the chemo in wheelchairs, and here's me complaining that I can't get out of bed for a few days.

But she is right, I do trivialise my illness; maybe that is one of the ways of coping with it. If I diminish its power over me as an illness, then it won't get the better of me. If I deny the seriousness of it and the intensity of it, then it will disappear, but like all demons in our life, the only way of dealing with them is facing them.

I have decided that I will make a New Year's resolution and that is to be kinder to myself. I am always so hard on myself and with what has happened to me it is time to stop that. I need to realise that I am vulnerable and I need people, and that I am not perfect. If I feel upset and sad it is not a matter of shame to communicate it, and I've found that when you tell people you've been ill or that you are fed up, the whole world doesn't suddenly fall apart and some people actually say things that make you feel better or that you are not alone. All my life I have tried to take on the whole world by myself and it is a bloody big world to be able to keep that up for ever. So this year I will resolve to be kinder to myself.

January 9, Tuesday

Went to Welsh class today, the first time in three weeks. God, no wonder the language almost died out! It's so difficult! My fluency goal is now three as opposed to two years – if, in fact, that was ever my goal. Two years is laughable. I don't think I will ever get the hang of it, it's like learning Chinese. And Welsh speakers go on about how easy it is to speak. Of course it is for them – they were born speaking it! It is a language that is in the breastmilk of Welsh speakers: it has to be, to get your lips around the pronunciation.

Welsh is about these things called 'treiglads'; essentially, it makes the four die-hards left in our class recoil in horror every time we have to learn a new set of grammar rules – which is every lesson, as it is an intensive course. Treiglads are the Offa's Dyke of the Welsh language, only invented by Welsh speakers to keep even the keenest of English-speaking monoglots out. There are three different sets of treiglads and fifteen letters in the alphabet are affected by them. I asked Rhodri how many letters were affected by treiglads and he said, 'I don't know,' and that's even more infuriating as Welsh speakers who have heard the language since they were born didn't have to learn them and they are as natural as a hill or a stream or a bloody daffodil to them. Anyway it's very hard and not for the faint-hearted, but I will not be defeated by it, mainly because living in a house full of men speaking a different language to me is a treiglad too far.

Miss Fran, Elis's music teacher, came this evening and it has only taken two years for him to settle down to it. The thing is, I have slight guilt pangs about him playing the piano as it is something that I have wanted to do all my life. It's one of those 'living your unfulfilled desires through your children', things.

If my children show the slightest bit of interest in

anything, I'm there. That is probably because I myself was not wholly encouraged in things I liked – music and drama – so I grew up being shy and lacking confidence in my abilities. *Michelle lacks confidence in her own abilities* should be my bloody epitaph, it was written on so many school reports.

Elis is actually quite good on the piano. He can pick a tune up immediately by ear, much like I could when I was his age, and it's got to be in his genes with all Rhodri's family.

Sioned is a concert harpist, Rhodri has a music degree and lives his life with musical scores, and both he and his aunt agreed the piano was the instrument that Elis should learn, because that gives you a grounding in music for life. The lovely Miss Fran said he was very talented musically, and that you often found musical children were naughty. I didn't like to tell her it was probably a result of seven years of lackadaisical parenting.

Anyway she has persevered and he does seem to be getting there, also due largely to the fact that Miss Fran found a book called *Piano for the Young Football Fanatic* – what could be more perfect? I have asked him a few times if he wants to stop, but he doesn't, so he is getting something out of it. In a while, he will be able to read music; he will have achieved something and he won't feel, like I did, that he wasn't given the opportunity.

Practice with him is a little painful but we will persevere, get him through some exams and give him another language – music – that no one will be able to take away from him.

Rhodri came home about eight and we ate together for the first time in ages. I am getting a bit fed of being on my own but hey, *surra surra* (that can't be how you spell it, but *beth banneg*, as I have been saying in Welsh – whatever).

I made fajitas. God, I have put on so much weight over Christmas. I didn't eat well when the chemo knocked me out, and I just seem to have to put huge amounts of food away ever since. I know steroids do it, but I'm only on them for three days so I don't know if it works like that.

Also, I can't stop eating chocolate and there is loads of it in this house, and yet I don't really like chocolate. Actually, I only crave chocolate when my period is due, and I attribute this to lack of iron. Gill said my red blood count was down, so maybe it's my body's way of telling me I need iron – great justification for stuffing yourself with chocolate.

I am now taking a multivitamin with iron which is a bog-standard Tesco thing; in the Velindre booklet it says you can take them. I can't wait for my last chemo so that I can get on my mega-supplements and try to cleanse my body and build my immunity up again. Will start eating soups tomorrow, manyana manyana.

Rhodri and I watched *Bones* together. It's a forensic thing on Sky or, as Elis says when he sees these things on the Sky-plus planner, 'Mum, why do you always watch things with dead bodies in them?' Rhodri and I have become slightly addicted to it. I started watching it, now he wants to watch it too – foxy lead characters, eye candy for both of us, bit of sexual tension here and there and a corpse or two. What could be more perfect of an evening? What's more, husband and wife can immerse themselves in the world of forensic anthropology without ever having to give a thought to their own anthropological angst. Basically it means you can legitimately NOT talk to your partner for an hour and not be accused of not talking to your partner for an hour.

It's always slightly disappointing at the end though, because I usually know who has done it within the first ten minutes (I am a forensic/FBI genius and clearly wasted in the media), but it is always the person you do not expect. Although I was slightly flummoxed the other day when the doctor turned out to be the cannibal – hadn't seen that one coming at all.

Then I was going through the Sky planner and thought I'd watch a Christmas documentary I'd recorded on C.S. Lewis. This is part of a master-plan of trying to watch things slightly more worthy and educational than *Bones* – although if I did ever find a mummified body in the middle of nowhere, I would certainly know now not to contaminate the crime scene.

So we watched this documentary and I thought it was going to be this gentle romp through Narnia and him at Oxford and his idyllic upper-middle-class childhood, but oh my God I was SO wrong. At one point I was crying so much I was shaking, and I actually sobbed out loud. First his beloved mother, who was the centre of his universe, died of cancer leaving his bereft father unable to connect emotionally with his two small grieving children; he sent them away to boarding school.

Then C.S. Lewis's wife got cancer and died leaving *him* with two small step-children who had lost their mummy – the centre of their universe. He too was bereft and unable to connect with the grieving children, until the youngest boy hugged him and said 'What are we going to do now?'

It was heartbreaking – truly heartbreaking. I wanted to give all those little boys their mummies back to love them with all their hearts as it should have been.

When it ended, the actor playing C.S. Lewis turned to the viewer, reflecting upon the tragedies of his life, and said he likened his journey to that of the great lion Aslan in Narnia. They cut off Aslan's beautiful mane and sacrificed him, but the reality was that he came back stronger; that is what tragedy does to you, but if you look closely enough you just might see the scars. And I thought, What an amazingly powerful metaphor that was for someone who was battling, and winning their fight with cancer, as I hope I am.

For that is what it is, a battle, just like they faced in Narnia. Your mane is cut off, literally in the case of someone having chemotherapy when your hair goes, and with it some of your dignity is lost; you sacrifice some of yourself when you are weak but the sacrifice and the battle means that you come back stronger, like Aslan. I will try to remember to hold on to that.

January 10, Wednesday

Hurrah hurrah hurrah. I have booked a two-week holiday for the four of us in Menorca in May – sun, sand and kid's club, and, with a bit of luck, if I'm feeling up for it, sex and Sangria. It is half-board in a hotel, something we have never done before as we are normally 'independent travellers' which is short-hand for finding your own way from the airport, never being sure what standard your accommodation is, and not really having anyone to complain to when you get there if you need to.

It also means having to cook your own food and wash your own dishes (by hand) for two weeks because rustic cottages don't have dishwashers. You have to do this constantly because no sooner is one meal finished and cleaned away, you are washing dishes from the next one. So even though Rhodri was being VERY snobby about it, I have insisted we go in a hotel so that someone else is cleaning it for us, and half-board so I don't have to go anywhere near a sink OR spend my entire life looking for a restaurant that will cater for my finikity children's taste.

Usually this means spending twenty pounds on a meal for them they will not eat, because the pasta is not like the pasta they have at home, or the chips are the wrong shape or it has an onion in it or it is just plain 'yucky', as Osh likes to say. So someone else will provide the food and they must surely be well versed in catering for children. The children will have something to eat and, if we don't like it, which is unlikely in my case as I really will eat anything, we can go to a restaurant later in the evening after they have eaten.

I have a spring in my step today, something to look forward to after my treatment. Elis will have to come out of school for a week and I haven't asked them yet, but I'm sure I can fulfil their teaching objectives for the week – I never know exactly what he does there, so that might be quite illuminating in itself. When you are ill you can't imagine what it is like being well, and when you have spent an entire winter with torrential rain you cannot imagine what sunshine is like.

I am looking in the Next catalogue at chocolate-coloured kaftans and chocolate leather mules. I will be a vision in chocolate – let's hope I don't melt!

Went to see Rosie today and told her I was unwell after the last chemo. I asked if I could do a bit of an experiment and do three sessions before my next chemo instead of two. I want to see if this makes any difference because, if it does, it will at least stop me being in bed for four days. It's not just the being in bed, because it takes about a week to recover from being ill, as you're just not quite yourself. So I am having one next week and one the Monday before my next chemo. Fingers crossed it will work.

January 11, Thursday

Christine, Elis's childminder, has said she can't pick Elis up on Monday as she has to go to the hospital. She has had ovarian cancer and has had chemotherapy TWICE. She has been a great help to me as she knows what I am going through. She has had some problems and is getting it checked out. I have been thinking about her a lot recently. I am worried about how I will learn to live with having had cancer, and what would happen if it comes back. But these are a lot of ifs and buts and may never happen.

Gill says my chances of the cancer coming back would

be about one in eight, as opposed to the rest of the female population, which is one in nine, and I think they are very good odds, thank you very much. I will not be Googling anything that might tell me different.

For Christine, she has to live with the possibility of her cancer returning, and I have no idea how she does that. She is a great role model as she had cancer for a year and I didn't know about it until her hair fell out. She looks after Elis and the other children she picks up, with her husband's help, and always seems to have loads of energy. I am saying a little prayer for her that it is a blip and that everything will be OK.

January 12, Friday

Christine's daughter has had a baby boy: Oliver Samuel. I am so pleased Christine has something to take her mind off her troubles and that there is a new baby in the world. I have bought him a Noukie Paco. Osh has one of these permanently in his hand. It is a donkey's head on a little blanket (not the *Godfather*-type horse's head thing, something much softer and cuter). Joanne bought it for Osh when he was born and he took to it straight away. The only problem is, since Noukie version one I have spent over one hundred and fifty pounds on Noukies (all the same ones) as he has lost so many of them and he simply cannot live without it. It is a relationship I have only ever come across in Philip Pullman's book – Noukie is Osh's Daemon. They are as one. Except he's not the same one but Osh doesn't care or know this, apart from one Noukie which, out of all the many Noukies I have bought, he rejected and would have nothing to do with. All very weird. When Osh is parted from Noukie for a little while he is very twitchy about the whole business.

At one point he was losing one a week, usually in Tesco.

They NEVER had any of them handed in, which was a bit strange. I think there might have been a Noukie kidnapper in the store. I have several in the house at any given time in use and new ones in packets waiting to be used should any of those go AWOL. If Noukie gets lost, Osh will not go to sleep and whinges incessantly until he has him again. My mother lost one once when she was looking after him (he had actually put it in a vase and forgotten where it was) and she had to bring him back because he was crying so much. She also has a spare one up there permanently now.

Nigel has finished the shelves and the door and they look really lovely; they all need painting now. At the beginning of the week Rhodri said he would do them as I thought I wouldn't have the energy to do them myself, but now I feel as if I could do anything so have started undercoating the shelves so I can gloss tomorrow. House is in total chaos, need to restore order.

Elis had Ben around after school. I like him to have children around the house so that he can develop his social skills and basically leave me alone for a few hours on a Friday afternoon while I read the paper. Osh usually won't leave them alone, he's in the bedroom with them. In the winter they play FIFA 07 on the Playstation and in the summer they play football in the garden; either way it reinforces their male obsessive behaviour around sport which will no doubt stay with them for the rest of their lives, and all because I wanted five minutes' peace on a Friday. What *am* I doing for their future spouses?

Elis is going on a sleepover tomorrow at Jonah's house for Jonah's birthday. Nerys, Jonah's mother, has Jonah, Jay and Elis sleeping over, and Jonah's sister has her friend. I wish her good luck, that's all I can say. Having more than two of them in the house for small periods of time can be quite stressful and you find yourself arbitrating constantly. So, in light of the fact that Rhodri and I only have one wee small child left with us, who is very portable, I've invited ourselves over to Ian J's for a sleepover which he is all for – someone to cook for us, no babysitting fees and, more importantly, a few glasses of wine which I am really up for now.

January 13, Saturday

I woke at seven and started painting the shelves; I finished at one with only a short coffee break. It was very satisfying doing the job and they really do look lovely. I was a bit concerned they would make the room look too cluttered but I've de-cluttered the piano, which is a station for letters and correspondence we don't know what to do with, and have taken a rather busy rug off the floor and it looks really really nice. Front door also very nice.

Osh's bedroom is over the front porch and there was only a thin piece of board between the floor and the outside world so it is no wonder it has been so cold in there; that's why we had the outer door put on, all very plain, simple, and tasteful of course.

I snuggled Osh up last night and I said, 'You're nice and cosy now, Osh, with your new windows and your new door keeping out the cold.' 'Yes,' he said, 'new windows and new doors in the bank's house.' He and Elis are always arguing about whose house it is. Osian says, 'It's Oshy's house,' and Elis says, 'It's my house,' and I say, 'no, it's the bank's house.' So Osh now calls everything the bank's. The bank's blue door, the bank's garden, the bank's windows. I would try to explain that we own a percentage of it but think that might be lost on him. I'll be putting our books on the bank's shelves tomorrow.

Dropped Elis off at Jonah's and decided to get Osh a haircut. He fell asleep in the car and stayed sleeping when I put him in his pushchair, for over an hour, so I nipped into a café and had a coffee and read a whole newspaper in one go without him waking – what bliss! Met Rhodri after the football match and we went home together and then on to Ian J's.

January 14, Sunday

We had a lovely evening at Ian J's, and needless to say drank far too much champagne. Ian likes his champagne and who am I to complain? I've always been a bit of a champagne socialist. I felt slight twinges of, 'Oh, I shouldn't be doing this,' but it's not as if I am drinking all the time, and the last time I had a hangover was eleven days ago, to be precise, and that would have been unheard of before I had cancer so I will bloody well pat myself on the back for being good.

I definitely need to give myself a break from my own constant criticism. Oh my God, is this what I am like with Rhodri? No wonder we have entered into an aggressive-defensive relationship.

Rhodri got all the books down from the attic and there's one called *Hot Buttons*; it's about how to resolve conflicts and calm everyone down. It's explores aggressive and defensive relationships – well, the bit I dipped into did anyway. And I thought, God, that *is* me and Rhodri: I'm aggressive about something and he is defensive, then I get aggressive about him being defensive and he is probably only defensive because he has lived for years with my bossy aggression. We so have to get out of this cycle. Correction, *I* have to get out of that cycle as I think I might be the cause in the first place.

Deborah would no doubt be proud of me, that I am realising that not everything is actually Rhodri's fault and maybe, just maybe, it might be something to do with me as well as him. I will work on that – I'll read on in *Hot Buttons* to see if I can get some 'tools' to resolve it.

We started putting books on the shelves and I am so glad we've got them down at last, not least because the damp was beginning to affect them. There's some lovely art and reference books and I was showing Elis loads of things when I suddenly realised I haven't read a book since *The Kite Runner*, other than self-help ones, which I never seem to finish. Mind you, *The Kite Runner* was so traumatic for me it's not surprising, but I do want to read again. I want to be able to discuss books and films, which I never go and see, and go to the theatre. When was the last time I went to the theatre?

I feel another belated resolution coming on. I will resolve to go to the theatre and cinema and basically take in a bit more culture. I am starting a diet tomorrow; I have been eating crap since Christmas, I cannot stop eating crisps, and if there is any chocolate anywhere near me, it's gone within minutes. I can feel I've put on weight, so I want to lose it before our sun-drenched holiday.

There is also one other reason for wanting to lose weight; namely, it is very difficult to pull off the Kylie-looking-fabulous-with-short-hair-look if you have a double chin. Kylie looked good in those headscarves – and believe me I have been around enough women cancer patients to know this is a very difficult look to pull off.

On me they look hideous, no matter what colour they are or how I tie them. They only just cover my head – as it is so big – and they just don't suit me. Now Kylie is elfin, she has the face and the features that can carry off a headscarf and the same beautiful face and features that can carry off that 'very short hair look' without people immediately thinking, Oh my God, that person has had cancer.

I think if you have very short hair and don't have the face for it, people think one of two things: cancer or lesbian. I have nothing against lesbians, who rank among some of my very good friends, but there is a stereotypical idea that they do go around with very short hair.

My hair is well over an inch in length, BUT it is very thin and mostly grey. I am hoping that when the chemo finishes, the bits without hair will start filling out and it won't be long then until I can take off my wig. It's one thing having very short grey hair, BUT having short grey hair AND being fat is really not the post-cancer look I was aiming for.

I am thinking more fragile and beautiful but radiant at the same time – in fact, I have just described Kylie. Although my wig has been very good for me, I really do want my hair back. I keep dreaming that I wake up and I can comb my own hair. I don't really mind about it being short and I will put a henna dye on it – as you can't use any other dye.

I figure very short hair and very bright lipstick. Bright lipstick covers a multitude of sins. I will treat myself to one of those expensive designer ones that stay on all day, even in a force ten gale.

Rhodri is doing a documentary on jazz musician Al Bowlly – I have never heard of him – and has been thinking of angles to approach him. That's what you do in documentary-making, well, that's what you are supposed to do but I have worked in the industry long enough to know that some people still don't have a bloody clue. If you find yourself switching over when you are watching one, it is usually because there is no narrative to the documentary. Anyway, I have done some internet research on him for Rhodri as I was bored and I used to be a researcher and want to impress my husband with factoids I have gathered. Dennis Potter was influenced by Bowlly, who died in the London Blitz in 1941. The upshot of my research is that I have felt my brain is stirring and getting into gear, and I have found work can be quite interesting. So I have Al Bowlly and Rhodri to thank for that.

January 15, Monday

Saw Deborah this morning, my last appointment. I told her I hadn't had much time for existential angst as I had been too busy, and wasn't sure what I could talk about, forgetting completely that I had been ill and crying after my last chemo. Ah, the mind is a great healer. It also has a way of playing tricks on you because nine days ago I couldn't get out of bed and by now I had forgotten how that had made me feel.

I talked about getting on with my life; I felt I was ready to move on. She said (more or less) that I diminished my experiences often, and she is right: I always say there is someone worse off than me, someone with a worse cancer, or someone who has experienced terrible tragedy in their life, like the loss of a child, and that I feel that my suffering could not be on a par with that.

That does have some truth BUT she is also right that I do have a serious illness and I should be easier on myself. I suppose going to see her has made me understand how I have tried to trivialise my illness, and also, being so poorly after my last chemo, has made me aware that I am vulnerable and I need to confront the seriousness of what has happened to me.

There is a small dark place in my mind where this exists: the horrible truth of the enormity of having cancer. It is such a terrifying place that to visit and confront it in one go would have been too much for me. I have to open that door very slowly, and confront some of those feelings very slowly, but at least now I am opening the door.

I have asked Deborah if I can see her again in a few months. I think that she can help me a bit later on, when I have finished my treatment. I'll have had time to reflect upon things more then. In many ways I feel I have only begun to scratch the surface of my emotions and feelings; I want to make sure that I come out the other end of this with a more open mind, not one that I am closing down.

January 16, Tuesday

Welsh class today. I have done absolutely zero work for it, but have, however, decided to enter myself for the exam. It covers the first thirty units of the course (half of it) and you either have a pass or fail. I'm rather hoping it will be a pass. If I enter for the exam, it means that I will have to pull my finger out; actually sit down and learn the first thirty units and also go to two revision days. This way, I might begin to seriously apply myself to learning the language. Rhodri picked Elis up to do music practice and homework as Miss Fran is coming early tonight. It is painful to hear them – I know how dentists feel – it's like pulling teeth.

January 17, Wednesday

Had acupuncture with Rosie. My period has started a week early, so I'm now definitely all up the Swanee. It's beginning to get as bad as it was at Christmas, but it's not there yet. I'm hoping that that was a blip and this next one will not be as bad. Pip came round with a birthday present for me. She thought my birthday was the nineteenth, not the twenty-ninth; it was a faux-fur hot water bottle cover and hot water bottle – perfect.

Pip has been such a great friend throughout my illness. She knows when all my chemo sessions are, is always sending me little cards and bought me a token to go and have a facial; and now a lovely gift. It's funny because sometimes the people you least expect are the ones who are there for you. Not that I thought Pip uncaring, she is very caring, but it just shows the strength of her character that she remembers all the little things about my life and is always there. Like with Kerry, our friendship has grown so much. Kate, too; ironically enough, we have got closer since her divorce. Sarah my sister sent me this email about sisters in the sense of all women being sisters and how much you gravitate towards women as you get older. It's true, I used to have more menfriends than women.

I showed Kerry the poem and she said she used to have more menfriends than women too, but it slowly dawned on her that she was backing the wrong horse – we both laughed a lot over this.

Having cancer is a strange thing, because before I left work there were people who I could see actively avoiding me, and the thing is, you don't expect them to be gushing all over you, or even say anything at all, but when you can spot them tapping the button of the lift manically to try to avoid actually having to speak to you, it's rather amusing. You feel like saying, 'Don't worry, it's not catching!'

January 18, Thursday

Went out with Babs last night for a meal. I was so happy to be out of the house. I really am stir-crazy. I haven't been out for ages and I just go a bit mad, like I did at Ian J's on Saturday. Rhodri got up with the children and took them to school and I didn't get up until ten-thirty. It was bliss. The blissful feeling didn't last long though, for as I came downstairs I couldn't believe my eyes: there was water pouring in through the windows and dripping in several places on the ceiling, including through the light fittings. I got a pile of towels and bowls and was saying, 'Bloody hell!' every time I spotted a new minor disaster. I immediately rang the builder who did the extension. They already have to come back in the summer to redo the door, and now their bloody roof is leaking! They came to have a look, but the weather was so bad they couldn't go out. They are coming back to investigate when it has stopped raining. It is blowing a gale – next door and next-door-but-one's fences and wall have all blown down, like dominoes. After Richard, the builder, left, the rain stopped for about half an hour and I went out to investigate. Some tiles have blown off the roof, the guttering is gone and the water is running down the side of the house into a small crack on the extension, so it's not a dodgy extension, thankfully. Need to get a roofer to come out now.

Elis had a friend, Alex, round after school. Elis seems to think it is his duty to tell his friends that his mother is wearing a wig. I am not sure why, maybe in case it accidentally blows off, revealing me to be the bald impostor I really am. Alex was pointing at things like a chair or Scooby Doo and was asking Osh what they were, because last time he saw Osh, he couldn't say that much. And Elis points to my head and says, 'Osh, what's that?' And he goes to Alex, 'It's a wig Alex. My mother wears a wig,' and continued to stress it about three times. Last time Ben, his other friend, came and we were sat at the dinner table, Elis said, 'Why don't you take your wig off, Mum?' Luckily Elis's friends don't seem to take any notice.

January 19, Friday

I must be mental taking the Welsh exam, even though the teacher keeps stressing how 'easy' it is. You do have to know your treiglads and they are the work of the devil. I have not really worried that much about treiglads as I feel they will spontaneously come to me one day, but now I have to sit down and learn the bloody things. Not quite sure why I am giving myself this extra bit of stress in my life but I suppose it is a very good focus and will take my mind off impending radiotherapy. I really will have to do a concentrated bit each day.

Went to see Elis in a concert at school. His class were all playing recorders – together they sound almost bearable. He was practising at home and I said, 'Now do it properly,' thinking he was messing about and he said, 'That was properly.'

I know it's a cliché but it sounded just like someone murdering a cat. I am outwardly supportive of his recorder practice, but it is the sort of sound that really grates on my nerves. I knew that when Rhodri suggested he play it.

I met Alison K after the concert and she told me that her father has cancer – he was perfectly well one minute and the next minute they found out he had cancer. Cancer creeps up on you, it is a law unto itself. I would not have known I had cancer until it had spread, quite possibly to my other organs or until it was so big I could actually feel it, unless I had had that mammogram. It is a slow silent killer.

My grandmother had a cancerous lump weighing two pounds removed from her chest when she was in her seventies and she lived another sixteen years after that.

Alison K looked very pale. I think she is the person in the family who has to hold it all together. I said to Rhodri that we will all be there one day (meaning with major illnesses); it is just a horrible thought that you have to face these things. Then I thought, What am I talking about? I am facing it, I am there. But I guess I also mean with our parents we will become the ones who take control, that role reversal when the child becomes the parent and your mother and father let you take over because they no longer have the energy to be the parent. You suddenly have to be both child and parent at the same time; it is a heartbreaking role as you grieve for the parent and you grieve for the child.

January 20, Saturday

Rhodri took Elis to football this morning. It has at least stopped raining temporarily. We had a pizza last night and I had cava, I managed not to drink an entire bottle, there was about half a bottle left – result. Rhodri said he thought that I should not be drinking at all when I was on chemotherapy, which I did not want to hear but I did ask him the question. It's the old story – ask him a question and he gives the answer I don't want to hear, then I get nasty with him. I guess I have married my conscience, because he never says the thing I want to hear. I know that when I ask him something, he will give me the answer that is unspoken in my own head, but when he does, I blame him for it. So essentially I am blaming him for the things I feel that I should not be doing. He really is in a no-win situation, for he doesn't realise that in speaking the truth, he's on to a permanent bloody loser.

I will resolve not to ask Rhodri the questions to which I know I will not like the answer.

If I wish to have a drink, I must take that responsibility upon myself and not blame Rhodri for what I perceive to be my failings. If I don't perceive them to be failings, I should savour the two glasses of cava, realise that life is very short and make the most of it, instead of arguing with my husband who let's face it has to put up with me. I must be a real pain in the arse to live with even when I haven't got cancer, so God knows what I'm like when I have.

I think that having cancer has a similar effect on your marital relationship as having a baby. Spending that stressful time together in all its goodness and all its badness makes you come out the other end a stronger couple – or you split up.

I thought that Rhodri was the one who had to grow up – and he did, he has – but it turns out I also have a bit of growing up to do. That never changes because each part of our lives, each new challenge we encounter, becoming parents, our illnesses, our parents' illnesses, the twists and turns in our relationships, mean that we are growing up all the time. I just want to make sure that Rhodri and I will do our growing up and growing old together.

January 21, Sunday

Rhodri and Elis have invited Jonah and Jay around to watch Man U v Arsenal. I have decided that there will be too much testosterone in the house for me and Osh, and am taking him to visit my mother. I guess this is it now, I am resigned to a life with a house full of men (well, boys at the moment, but they will turn into men) who are shouting at a television screen while thirty (not sure how many men make up two football teams, but I think it is fifteen each side) kick a ball around until one team wins or draws. I am looking on the bright side though, as it means I can just go shopping by myself for the next twenty years, now that my life has been saved.

January 22, Monday

My last chemo is due next Wednesday and in my mind that has already happened. I cannot wait to be free of it – I will put up with the side-effects if I have to be in bed for four days, but I'm having acupuncture with Rosie tomorrow to see if it makes any difference. If not, I'm thinking, That's OK – four days in bed and I never have to have it again. I want to be able to say, 'That's it, it's done,' but there is a nagging part of my mind, a tiny little bit, that says otherwise. There is a dichotomy going on in there, a little dialogue. It goes something like this. One bit says, 'I'll never have to have chemotherapy again, hurrah, this is my last session, I am free.' The other little bit of my mind says, 'Hang on a minute. Don't get too cocky because you know people who have had to have it twice, and if you are too cocky it might come back and that would be your own fault because you were so happy that it was over that you brought it back yourself.'

So part of me wants to jump up in the air and scream, 'Thank God that is over!' but the other part of me says, 'Be quiet! And if you are quiet and still and small enough, it might just forget you are there and not come back again.'

I will definitely have to see Deborah again in a few months and tell her this, as I worry, not only about this internal dialogue, but that there is a cancer type. I think I am a cancer type, as I worry about everything, and as much as I am trying not to be like this, I am essentially Chicken Licken. I think that this constant worry inside and never getting it out, that jolly cancer victim, is an unhealthy place to be. Those things can eat away at you, and I need to have some kind of balance in my mind instead of being constantly afraid that the cancer might come back because I drank some wine or because I ate some red meat. I am forgetting my 'be kind to myself' motto already.

January 23, Tuesday

I was feeling a bit demob happy at coming to the end of my treatment, but there's always someone ready to 'piss on your chips' as they say in the valleys. I went for blood tests today and my blood count was down so I need to have them done again tomorrow. Then I thought I would see Gill as usual and have a chat about how I was feeling, but saw another nurse and a pharmacist who came in to discuss the radiotherapy and Tamoxifen, so was a bit overawed by that.

They asked me if I had any worries and I told them that I had noticed some discharge coming out of my nipple (not the one I had the surgery on). They said it was impossible for a tumour to grow while having chemo, but they would get a doctor to examine me.

I discussed ovary removal with them and asked what their thoughts were, and they said I needed to discuss it with the doctor. Then Gill came in and said they could refer me to a gynaecologist; I was starting to get a bit freaked out by this time, as it was too much info to take in, in one go.

They enquired why I wanted my ovaries removed and I said I was terrified of getting pregnant and that if I did, it would boost oestrogen in my body. Gill said it would not make the cancer grow, but I am always sceptical about that, even though I am, of course, not medically trained. I read in Susan Love's book that it can take a cancer six years to grow to 1.5 cm – the size of my tumour – so that could have been the time I had Elis. Even though this might not be medically correct, it's in my mind now; it could be nonsense but I see oestrogen as a source of evil for me, and want it out.

Then they talked about osteoporosis and said that it shouldn't affect me because I have a healthy diet, etc. A female doctor whom I haven't met before came in to talk me through the radiotherapy and to get me to sign the consent form.

Firstly she examined my nipple, and said, 'Oh yes, I can see where that discharge is coming from. I'll speak to Dr Barrett-Lee, but I am not worried about it.' That is easy for her to say. The last time I was told I had nothing to worry about, I had a cancerous tumour. She came back and said they'd do a mammogram a few months earlier than the one scheduled in August, just to dot the i's and cross the t's – which again is fine for her to say, but means I will exist in a permanent state of anxiety until then. She talked me through the radiotherapy saying that at the moment, with a lumpectomy, the chances of that cancer returning were 20 per cent; with radiotherapy and Tamoxifen the chances went down to 2 per cent, which is the same odds as someone having a mastectomy but they have preserved the breast – good news so far.

'What if the cancer comes back?' I asked. 'Will you just take it out again and will I have chemo and radiotherapy again?'

'Yes, if we can take it out.' She was reading through my notes and said, 'You had an aggressive cancer and pre-cancer,' which was the first time I have heard about the pre-cancer or certainly registered this.

I asked her to explain what that meant, but I was not really taking it in and wished there was someone else with me to remember some of this. She said the excellent news was that it had not gone to my lymph glands, because they are the gateway to the rest of the body, but that basically there was a chance that it could spread to other organs, like the liver or bones or lungs. They will monitor me for the next five years to make sure that it doesn't come back in my breast and that my other organs are not affected.

I was in mild shock by this time. She asked me if she had explained properly and I said, 'Yes. I am just wondering how I will live for the next five years, thinking about this.' She said I would learn to forget about it and probably, when my next appointments were due, I'd worry about it, but no more than anyone else sitting out in that waiting room.

That didn't help me when I was in a state of mild meltdown, so I left feeling as if someone had punched me in the stomach and that I had been diagnosed all over again. I now have to think about liver cancer and bone cancer and lung cancer and brain cancer and osteoporosis and having my ovaries taken away and the side-effects of Tamoxifen and early mammograms, and it is so much information I think my head is going to explode.

So I get home and I call Rhodri and ask him to come home from work immediately, which he does, no questions asked. Luckily he is in Cardiff, as coming home from Spain could have been a bit tricky. When he gets in, I am sobbing uncontrollably because I don't want to die. I said that I felt guilty because I was happy it was going to be over soon and that I shouldn't be so happy in case something happened and this has happened because I was feeling so happy and believing that I would never ever have to think about cancer again, but I was wrong. Cancer is going to be there, hanging over me like a dark shadow, and I don't know how it will ever go away.

January 24, Wednesday

I went to see Rosie yesterday afternoon. She said she would get my blood count up as it was down, and she has; it has shot up – she's a miracle worker. Rhodri came to the hospital with me. This was it – the last appointment. I have never been so glad to get something over with in all my life. I feel physically sick writing about it, and every time I think about the place I feel an urge to throw up. I pray to God that I never have to go there again.

January 25, Thursday

Was very tired yesterday afternoon and I've been sleeping most of the day today, but I do feel much better than last time, so I do think the acupuncture is the key. I could not open my eyes last time I had chemo but now I am OK. As long as I rest, I can potter about the house and load the dishwasher and sweep the floor which would have been impossible last time.

Spoke to Sarah last night in Ireland – she is a born counsellor, that woman. I said I hadn't thought about the cancer coming back and all of a sudden I felt as if I had just had the diagnosis all over again , and I didn't want to die and I didn't want to think about cancer for the rest of my life. She said that it is better to acknowledge the fear and get it out there and deal with it, than leave it hiding somewhere.

I know she is right. I have to get this out of my system, I have to think it through. I am thinking about my life and how it will be, and whether I need to see Deborah again to talk through some of these dark fears.

I have been online and ordered some self-help books on living with cancer – the self-help industry is doing very well out of me at the moment – to get some perspective on it all.

Had to go to bed by eight as I was so tired. Rhodri came in about ten and brought me a tiny cake with a heart on it for Dydd Santes Dwynwen (the Welsh St Valentine's Day) and we ate some together. We lay together in the dark holding each other and I said, 'I don't want to die, I want to live with you and my babies and be happy,' and he said, 'You will be happy and you won't die,' and I believed him because I wanted to.

January 26, Friday

Julia and Joanne came down today for lunch. I am feeling so much better than last time, still tired but normal. I have stopped taking my tablets today – this is the earliest I have done this. Partly because I think they contribute to my general feeling of tiredness and I'd rather put up with feeling a bit sick, which isn't major. I am drinking Milk of Magnesium and Gaviscon and for me they work as effectively as the tablets do. I also want to stop taking them as it is one more step to being free of the chemotherapy.

I have been carrying around in my bag the little yellow card from the hospital which reads *I am a chemotherapy patient* and tells people what to do in an emergency, so I took it out of my bag and tore it into little pieces. I am no longer a chemotherapy patient. I will try to be strong and remember that, although I live with uncertainty, as Julia says, we all live with uncertainty – though it's not quite the same. I went to my friend Sarah's house the other day and a friend of hers was there whose son's schoolfriend had recently been killed. He was fifteen and had been knocked over – and I thought, God, you teach them over and over again that the road is dangerous, let them go slowly bit by bit when you can trust them, and then that happens and you wonder how you can live with it.

The mother had told Sarah's friend that she felt lucky because she had had him for fifteen years. I could not think of a more noble statement – that celebration of life in the midst of tragedy.

I suppose what I am afraid of is not the cancer coming back but dying and what death will be like; that may be morbid but I have to acknowledge those feelings. I must read *The Tibetan Art of Living and Dying* because I need to be spiritually uplifted and realise that death is inevitable, and that when my time comes I should be happy in my heart that I loved and was loved, and that would be enough for me.

January 27, Saturday

Why oh why am I doing this Welsh exam! I keep thinking I've got enough going on in my head without the added stress of learning where to mutate treiglads. I have spent all day thinking I should do it, but not even picking up a book, so then I think it was a mistake and I can't do it. And then I think that I desperately need another focus other than bloody cancer, so I will do it and have a go. I have almost three months to crack it, after all. I will start tomorrow.

Rhodri is in London and my mother has had the children; I've been out and about shopping and I feel a bit worn out now. I am forgetting that it was only Wednesday that I had my last session but feel so much better than the other times. I just want to be out there living my post-chemo life.

I have decided to try to be teetotal. Every time I drink now, I think about the physical effects. Wine gives the body an oestrogen boost, plus I want a pure clean liver. I have always thought that I need alcohol to have a good time, as I am essentially very uptight and it completely loosens my inhibitions, but if that is the case then something else in my life needs addressing.

I have been practically teetotal over the last few months anyway, so it's one step further. It's easy to think like this now as I have just had chemo and won't feel that well really for at least a week to ten days. After that, the old feelings of wanting to curl up with a bottle of wine and watch the telly or having friends over may creep back in. I will not say I will never drink again, but I am endeavouring not to drink on a regular basis. My theory is that I will immerse myself in Welsh and books, and write a novel or something and will forget alcohol.

I have become very sentimental about my husband – I think I have realised just how much I love him. My mother sent him a note on Friday with a bottle of wine (he also got a bottle of wine from my sister – he appears to be benefiting from my lack of drinking). The note said how proud she was to have him as a son-in-law and how grateful she was that he was there for me and to look after me. I read it and cried; of course, he had a tear in his eye too.

I have spent so much time thinking about myself throughout all this that I forgot to think how he might be feeling; part of me is frightened to acknowledge that he might be frightened too, because if he is, who the hell is going to look after nutty me when I have my meltdowns.

I was putting some socks in his sock drawer later when I was by myself and found a leather photo album that I put together about four years ago when he went off for five weeks working in America. It contains photos of me and Elis. The day after Rhodri left for his trip, I found out I was pregnant with Osh. I didn't tell him for about two weeks because I thought I was going to have a miscarriage, but it all worked out in the end.

I was looking through the album and thinking how much Osh looked like Elis, and spotted a wonderful black-and white-photo that Pip had taken of us on our wedding day. We look so young and beautiful and we look so much in love. I sat down and cried for that time when nothing had touched our lives. I have my head on his shoulder and am looking at him and he's talking to someone, drinking wine, and I looked at that photo and thought we were different people then, because nothing really touches your life in the way that cancer does.

We had Elis later and of course a child shapes and changes your life, but even though having a baby is a thunderbolt in some ways, a lot of changes are also gradual. Here we are: in the space of eight months our lives have changed irrevocably. There is no going back.

I looked at Rhodri, all handsome and smiling and smart in his wedding suit, and he looked like a little boy. I thought, He has gone from a boy who could not answer his wife's cries in the night when she prayed not to die, to a man who can stand by her side and make her feel that no matter what has been or what is to come, they will face it together. I am so absorbed in my own journey, I haven't noticed he's been on one too.

I took the photo out of the album and have put it in a frame on the piano, for even though we were different people then, that love still stands, more than ever.

January 28, Sunday

No Rhodri, no children last night. Home alone was VERY
WEIRD. Kept thinking all evening I would go up to the
farm and see them, but I was really very tired. When I was
putting clothes away in the boys' rooms and saw their little
empty beds, I wanted to drive up to the farm and grab hold
of them both and hug them until I couldn't hold them any
more. Tomorrow I will be forty.

Went up to the farm this morning to get my two little
monkeys and guess what – I was met with a surprise Happy
Birthday 40 Tomorrow party with fab presents and Joanne
and Russell, Julia, Emily, Mum, Dad, Janet and my Uncle
Ian and the children; it was really nice.

I had made Rhodri promise on pain of death that he
wouldn't do any surprise parties because I would not be
able to stand it. I had neglected to tell my family this,
however, as I thought it would be too emotionally
overwhelming but they did it and it was really lovely. I had
designer sunglasses and a bag from Julia and Martin and
Lloyd, a leather pouch full of Clarins make-up from my
Auntie Janet and my Uncle Ian, a fantastic necklace from
Joanne, Russell and Megan. Emily, Sarah and Aidan and
the boys have paid for flights to Ireland, and my parents
gave me Marks & Spencer vouchers and have paid for my
car-hire to Ireland and petrol. I felt like a WAG. It was all
beautiful stuff which everyone had put loads of thought
into. So I have already broken my teetotal rule and had a
glass of champagne. Well, you're only forty once and I'm
bloody glad I'm here to celebrate it!

January 29, Monday

They say life begins at forty and I am proceeding on that
basis. My star sign, courtesy of the *Daily Mirror* for 29

January, my forty-first year of existence, reads thus:

Perhaps certain dreams are gone for ever but still you must appreciate what you do have. The Sun's meeting with Chiron brings an opportunity for healing and the chance to build a new future. A new era is beginning and you need to play your part in what is created.

January 30, Tuesday

We took Osh and Elis out to a Chinese restaurant yesterday. I wanted a take-away then thought, No, we'll go out en famille so we'll all be at Mummy's fortieth birthday party. At the end of the meal Rhodri said, 'Thank God we only have to do that once every forty years.'

Basically, between the ages of one and four, children and nice restaurants don't really go together. Elis is OK but he did spill two full glasses of water over the table. Osh managed to snap BOTH chopsticks in half and constantly wanted to make a run for it, so you spend most of the meal telling him to sit down as, 'The man is watching' or 'A policeman is coming', which has little effect on him because he is two and why would he give a shit about the 'man' or a policeman?

We came back and Alison K was here with a bouquet of flowers and stayed for a bit. I had six bouquets of flowers delivered yesterday and even more fabulous presents. I have already broken my teetotal rule two days in a row, but, after all I have had *two* fortieth birthday celebrations. However, I only had a modest amount of wine and did not have a hangover this morning; a sure sign of my wisdom and maturity.

Managed to get Rhodri, for the first time I can remember in our ten-year relationship, to come to Marks & Spencer's – he didn't exactly embrace it with the enthusiasm that I apply to it, but he turned up and paid for the coffee.

Rhodri got a cake for me, with a photo of me and the boys on the top. Elis wanted to eat his face and Osian wanted to eat his face, so Rhodri and I had half each of my face. Rhodri is taking me away for a long weekend to Portmeirion in the next few weeks as a present. We went on honeymoon there and he is buying me a painting, but I haven't seen any I like yet.

Rhodri had also done an album for me: *forty photos for forty years*. It was a bit of a shock to see them all together because there is an image in my mind of a slim, tall, well-groomed woman. Basically that happened for about a two-year period in my life (between ten and twelve) and I am essentially a buxom wench and have never really been slim – it is pure fantasy. Instead of lamenting, I will embrace that image. After all, what the hell have I got to prove to anyone any more?

January 31, Wednesday

Had a facial today for the first time in my life. I don't know why I've waited forty years to do it, it was really relaxing. I don't really like massages and complete strangers touching me, but it was very nice. I've probably got over this because for the last eight months I have had to whip my top off and have men and women I have never met before, poking around my tits. The masseuse asked me if I could relax easily and I said not really. She also has two boys, a seven year old and a two year old, and we spent about fifteen minutes talking about what it is like. Her two year old is almost three, as well – all very spooky – and we both agreed that basically they left us exhausted but that they were lovely.

Anyway, she said, 'What do you do to relax?'

'Well, until recently I used to drink shedloads of alcohol,' (which she found very funny for some reason), 'but I am not doing that any longer, so I need to find other ways to relax. I am watching telly at the moment, and reading again.' This is a lie as I have not actually picked up a book yet but in my mind I am almost there. Self-help books are piling up by the side of my bed and I need to at least have a cursory glance at those before I move on to proper literature (at a rough count, I have about nine of them – think I might need to put them on a shelf somewhere as having nine self-help books, which includes *The Tibetan Book of Living and Dying*, is a little daunting). If they are on a shelf they will be less intimidating than sitting by the side of my bed, taunting me to help myself.

I am only just getting over the fact that I am coming out the other end of all this and I haven't had the radiotherapy yet. My Uncle Ian has had radiotherapy. He says it is fine and not to worry about it, which is good coming from someone who has actually had it, rather than my mother telling me about Mrs Jones's cousin's uncle's daughter who was fine.

For my mother, everything is fine because that is her way of dealing with life. I am trying not to fall into that trap. For instance, when I was talking to Kerry about Felix having tests for his leg, which aches, it would have been quite dismissive to say it would be fine, when I didn't know anything about it. Surely it is more sensible to say, 'You'll feel better when you've gone though all the tests and you know what the outcome is.' (I am a born therapist.)

I spoke to Karen in my Welsh class. Her sister-in-law died of breast cancer, and she asked me how I was doing. I said I had had a bit of a meltdown. She said you can't live your life thinking about what might happen to you; you need to go forward being positive.

I told her that in my head I had done cancer, cancer was there behind me and I wanted to go forward, but part of me is terrified of what might be. She said we can all be terrified of what might be, that anyone could have anything wrong with them, at any time, but that they can't live their lives thinking they will die, and that I am in a better place than most people, because I will be monitored for the next five years.

I am coming to terms with the fact that it is OK to think that I have done cancer, and to be positive about living my life. I saw the programme on Mr Monypenny that the BBC did. He is Mr Fantastic, and I can completely understand why, on all those soaps and American TV programmes, everyone falls in love with their doctors. I can imagine that Mr Monypenny would take you somewhere really nice for dinner, and know all about wine and would pull your chair out when you sat down. Mind you, I'd settle for a Harry Ramsden's in Cardiff Bay if he was sitting opposite me with his lovely, reassuring, smiley face.

Anyway, it showed him performing a mastectomy on a woman and I watched it and it made me feel much better to see a sentinel node being chopped up and analysed under the microscope. The woman who had the mastectomy said she felt 'lucky'; exactly as I have said many times. It is a word that people find very hard to associate with having cancer. She felt lucky that she would be able to live her life now, having caught the cancer early, and be with her children and grandchildren, and I thought it is very simple for her – she had negative nodes too, so that was very good news.

Kerry also had a facial after me and I looked after baby Daisy – she will go to anyone. I had to go to the supermarket to get Daisy some more milk, as I used Kerry's only bottle (I never listen to instructions), and I was in Tescos zipping about getting stuff for supper and I thought, Something's not right. I feel different – am I ill? Then I realised that for the first time in God knows how long, and I am talking years here, not just since my diagnosis, I felt relaxed. I was not tired, I was not sick, I was not anxious about what has been or what will be; for that moment in time, I was calm and relaxed as it should be, and I will NOT let cancer stop me feeling like that.

February 1, Thursday

Mowed the lawn today and trimmed the bushes; I really need to do more exercise, as I am becoming a slug. I figure the garden can benefit from my need to get up off my arse and lose a few pounds, so that I will be thin and gorgeous in a swimming suit when we go to Menorca.

People will, no doubt, look at me and marvel at the fact that I have two children and am so slim and trim. This is my fantasy, as is having hair and a figure like the post-cancer Kylie Minogue. She is my role model, and probably that of about fifty million other people – and that Oliver Martinez is a bloody fool. I do feel an affinity with her which is a bit ridiculous as we do have rather different lifestyles, but I think with breast cancer, or with any suffering, you can identify with people and it cuts across divides. Oh yes, I do love Kylie.

February 2, Friday

We are in Brighton, hurrah! I have managed to escape Cardiff and Wales and am on a mini-break – Bridget Jones style, except I have two children here too. We are at Ben and Bree's wonderful flat which is near Brighton Pier, overlooking the sea.

February 3, Saturday

The weather is glorious. There is a fair on the Pier, a park right by the house, mini-golf and the sea. Elis is in heaven –

mini-golf is his life. We haven't seen Ben, Bree and baby Nancy for six months but it feels like we saw them yesterday. I drank far too much wine and champagne last night (well, they had to celebrate my fortieth birthday) and am hungover today, but have walked miles as penance. Teetotalism has gone out the window but I don't really drink that much at all now so I'll stop beating myself up over the occasional drink. What is that old saying? 'If you give up drinking and you give up smoking and you give up sex, you won't live longer – it will just feel like it.' I realise that is not true, of course.

February 4, Sunday

Another glorious day – the sun always shines on the righteous. Baby Nancy is unwell, I think she's teething so Ben stayed in with her while, Rhodri and I, Elis and Osh and Bree went to the Brighton Pavilion, which was spectacular, if a little opulently OTT. We had those guides that are like phones, and Elis had one and listened to it all the way around really enjoying it; he is a child genius with his interest in Regency architecture. At the end he was pestering me to buy him a fan with a Chinese Dragon on it, and when I asked him what he wanted it for, he said, 'To fan myself when I am hot, of course.'

February 5, Monday

Back in Cardiff, I did some serious retail therapy with Kerry and baby Daisy. Rhodri's third cousin Sarah has had a baby girl so it was another opportunity to buy cute baby girl outfits. We had some photos through and Sarah looks fabulous. That's what having a baby at nineteen does for you: you bounce back. She is very young, but no younger than my mother when she had a baby. Pop them out when you are young, I say.

I also bought some pink, pretty (yet a little bit slutty) underwear from Next with a voucher Rhodri's Auntie Pauline gave me for my birthday. On the way to Brighton I asked Rhodri if he had any condoms and he said he hadn't bothered because he knew there was no chance he would be getting any sex. I hadn't brought any either and I felt a bit sad that sex is not a part of our life any more; neither of us even thinks about it. I cannot remember the last time we had sex; my treatment has worn me down so that sex is the last thing on my mind.

So when I went to get the children a Burger King in the service station I bought a packet of condoms in the toilet (£3 a pack – a pound a shag) and gave them to him. He said, 'These will probably expire before we get round to using them,' so I bet him £10 that we would use them all by the end of February. Kerry said Rhodri will think it's his lucky day when she saw my underwear. I said he is so desperate for sex, he would do me in a pair of fat pants and a binliner. Rhodri saw the underwear and did get very excited, but I had bought the wrong size bra so will have to change it tomorrow.

February 6, Tuesday

I had sex with my husband. I had sex with my husband. Did my husband in my (one size larger) new underwear. Thank you to Auntie Pauline for the voucher and Next for the slutty underwear which re-ignited my love life. Rhodri now owes me £3.3333 (recurring). Have just realised I have turned myself into a prostitute with my bet. Only have another twenty-two days to collect the further £6.666 (recurring).

February 7, Wednesday

Martyn forgot my birthday – actually he didn't forget, he sent me flowers, but I think that was after he remembered. So he took me and Sian from work (as she hasn't seen me since Christmas) out for a posh lunch to French restaurant Le Gallois. Although I am only eating dust at the moment to get into my new swimsuit, I forgot that and had two beautiful, but small courses. Sian and Martyn told me all the gossip from work so I am well up to speed on it all. Sian said, 'Sorry, Shell, you probably don't care about any of this,' but I did because for once it was really nice to speak about something other than my illness; I realised that there is another world out there that I belonged to once. Someone new is joining our team and I said, 'Make sure they don't take my desk,' and was all territorial about my working space, which would have been unheard of even a month ago.

February 8, Thursday

It is snowing. Osh looked out of the window and said, 'My garden is snowing,' and Elis woke up, looked through the window and screamed at the top of his voice as if someone was murdering him, 'It's bloody, bloody, bloody brilliant.' Osh has never seen snow; I think it has snowed once in his lifetime but he was tiny so he couldn't really remember it. Elis just wants to throw snowballs at everyone and make snow angels. Rhodri took them in the car to school; they were both so happy and excited to be out in the snow. As Rhodri pulled off, Elis had his head out of the window, his face beaming, catching the snow on his tongue and it was bloody, bloody, bloody brilliant.

Rhodri was supposed to be going to London today to queue in the American Embassy for a visa. He isn't going now because of the snow, so it means he can come to the hospital with me for my radiotherapy planning appointment, which I am glad about because I don't really want to go on my own. Also, if someone else is there and you ask questions, they can remember some of the good bits to counter-balance the bad bits which I tend to focus on at these times.

It's taken forty years, but I finally have a tattoo. We walked into the hospital and I said to Rhodri, 'I hate the smell of this place,' and he said, 'Oh, it's not that bad.' I don't think he can appreciate what the smell of the hospital does to me.

For the planning session, they lay you on a bed in the room and you have your top half bare, then they put these pen marks on you (not very high-tech, but I am assuming they know what they are doing) and then the bed moves through a piece of equipment which is like an enormous doughnut. It is very much like the Stargate in *Stargate*, or whatever it is called on Sky, but smaller, which was what I was thinking as I lay there, passing through the Stargate, bare-breasted with three blokes and a woman I have never met before, in another room watching me. Maybe it was one great big joke and the Stargate was actually real and I would be transported to another world or planet or back to June last year where they could undo my cancer diagnosis. This did not actually happen though.

Then this young lad came out and said, 'I am going to tattoo you now.' I wondered if he went down the pub after work and talked to his mates about what he'd done at work that day. Rhodri had suggested in the waiting room that I have *Bluebird* tattooed on it – a reference to Cardiff City and to the fact that my breast is still blue from the substance they injected into it when I had my first operation. (Or 'nuked me' as I say, but I have read on Google that it is not nuclear, although the sign on the door says *Nuclear Medicine*, so maybe I have that wrong.)

Then the young man tattooed three tiny dots on me and that was it. I had asked if I could see my consultant Mr Barrett-Lee, or Gill, as there were some questions I had to get out of my head or they would drive me crazy. Lizzie came, as Dr Barrett-Lee and Gill were out, and I asked her if I could have my mammogram soon to check out the nipple discharge, which I still have – even though it is a tiny amount. They have said it is nothing to worry about, but I am still worrying. If I were able to eliminate the worry from my mind with the mammogram, it would be great.

She said she would ask the doctor and come back to me. I also said that the costochondritis was back, which wasn't an issue, but I was scared in case it wasn't that but the cancer spreading to my liver, as I had read in Dr Susan Love's *Breast Book* that that is where you feel the pain for liver cancer. And even though that might be a mad thing to say, it was in my head and I'd feel better if it wasn't in my head but out there for someone to tell me it wasn't true.

She said that throughout my treatment my vital organs are monitored through my blood. I don't know how this is done, but I am willing, on this one, to take her word for it. She said that they would have been alerted to any change. They will continue to monitor me, and that if I had secondary liver cancer they would know about it. Hurrah! Someone in the medical profession has given me something concrete. Thank you, Lizzie, for putting my mind at rest.

I also asked about the chemo and would it now be out of my system, which she said it would be, but I might carry on feeling tired for a while. My immune system would be going up and up, and would soon be just like anyone else's.

So I was happy about that. I have decided not to take any of my boosting vitamins until after the radiotherapy, just my Tesco multi-vitamins and my Vitality with pro- and pre-biotic and omegas; then after the radiotherapy I will be back on the vitamin C and garlic and milk thistle and fish oils, and will read up on the others for long-term use.

I was reading an article in Rosie's waiting room on Allicin garlic. It is hailed as a wonder drug, so I will be taking that and vitamin C and the fish oils for the rest of my life – long may that be.

February 9, Friday

The snow is clearing. I did a bit of mad cleaning this morning. One of the reasons I will be glad to get back to work is that it will actually stop me cleaning, which I am slightly obsessive about. I guess it is the valleys girl in me. There it is seen as a reflection on you, how often you clean your front step.

It takes me an hour after Rhodri and the boys have left in the mornings just to get the house square, and then there's washing and bits of shopping and God knows what else. I have just got the Johnson's cotton buds out and have cleaned the glass door of the shower; I think it's turning into a bit of an addiction.

I long to be like the women whose houses I go to. These houses are not immaculate – I don't mean the toys on the floor, that's inevitable – but may have a dirty sink with bits in it that no one seems to notice, bits of food waiting to germinate into something hideous that would almost certainly wipe out my entire family. People whose houses have never seen a Johnson's cotton bud in the shower tray – how do I become one of those people?

How the hell did I manage to fit all this in before? Did I just not notice, or was I really Superwoman doing all this cotton-bud cleaning and working almost full-time, or was it a mess and I just didn't notice? Or I *did* notice but didn't care, or I *did* notice and *did* care and thereby worried myself into a life-threatening illness.

I'm trying to plough through my self-help books to justify the amount of money I have spent on them. There is one called *Cancer Positive* and it is really good, mainly because it is quite short which means I can read it twice to fully take it in. It is very reassuring to read, because many of the things the author says in his book, about changing your life, and how a diagnosis of cancer affects you and makes you re-evaluate your life, are the things that I have come to understand and appreciate.

There is mention in the book about 'the cancer type', although he may not actually say that; instead the author discusses how stress affects the immune system. The fact is I worry about mould (green and black) in the shower tray, and have to clean it out with a Johnson's cotton bud.

I have to let go of my worry. It has been programmed into me by my Auntie Beatty and my grandmother, who spent most of my childhood predicting terrible things would happen if I ran or climbed or ate lying down or was left in water too long, and I am exactly like them.

I was reading in the self-help section of Borders, when I went shopping with Kerry, another book – which I didn't dare buy, otherwise self-help will be becoming an obsession, and that will be another thing to worry about – but it was about a woman talking to another woman about worrying about her children. I thought, It's one thing to say, 'Let go of that anxiety and tension, the worrying that something might happen to them,' but how the bloody hell do you do that?

Isn't it programmed into us to be terrified that something will happen to our children, so that we are constantly looking out for them and making sure they stay alive? Isn't that a 'continuation of the species' thing, because if you didn't have a society full of completely paranoid mothers making sure their children lived to adulthood to reproduce, wouldn't society just end, crumble into dust?

If I wasn't worrying about the bacteria in the shower tray being potentially harmful to my children, wouldn't I be doing society and the whole human race a disservice?

February 10, Saturday

Weighed myself in Tescos; I have put on thirteen pounds. I am eleven stone thirteen pounds and I want to be back at eleven stone. When I met Rhodri I was about nine and a half stone. I have a big job to stick to eleven stone, so I must have been like Kate bloody Moss then. I was a vegetarian, rode a bike everywhere as I didn't have a car, and went swimming nearly every morning before work. HELLO – was I mad? Probably, but I was thin. Despite my 'I don't care what I look like as long as I am alive' mantra I really do want to lose that weight. I have a tartan mini-skirt which I don't dare wear until I am thinner, because I think I will be mutton dressed as lamb. But by then it will be summer and I'll have to wear it next winter now. The plan is to try and lose two pound a week. That should be possible, with lots of water and apples and soup.

February 11, Sunday

Went swimming with Elis this morning. I can't remember the last time I did that and it was great. Because he can swim now it means I am not sticking to him like a limpet, but can let him move around on his own and have races with him. I am determined to do some exercise. I feel like I've been hibernating since my diagnosis, not doing much of anything, just tied to the house.

Not having hair is also very liberating, as when you have hair you have to dry it and do stuff to it. My hair is starting to come back, I think I can see tiny little shoots on my head now where the patches were.

I was in a private cubicle with Elis and he was saying, 'Tell me when you are taking your wig off. I don't want to

225

look,' and he was making a fuss about it. I got cross and said, 'If you want to come swimming with me you will have to see me without my wig.' (I wore a swimming hat – very fetching, NOT; it was orange and I looked like an overweight Belisha Beacon.) Eventually he peeled his hands away from his eyes before I put the swimming cap on and he went, 'Hmm, it's not that bad, what are you worrying about?' as if he was about thirty, not seven. Then he completely ignored it.

February 12, Monday

I have a new lease of life, not just because I have had a cancerous tumour removed and might live to tell the tale, and not only might I live to tell the tale BUT I have also analysed, deconstructed and am attempting to put back together the remnants of my life. No, it is something even more life-affirming and life-enhancing than that.

It is the discovery, after a few phone calls and a bit of research, that we can just about afford to buy a static caravan in Tenby. If you had told me ten years ago that this would be the focus of my entire life, I would have laughed; now the thought of having a static caravan to escape to at weekends and school holidays is filling my every waking thought: I can't stop thinking about it, and talking about it, except to my parents who will give me advice that I don't want. So I am being a big grown-up girl and, along with Rhodri, as he is the one who has to pay for it, we are going to buy one, just like that. I feel as if I have just started an illicit love affair that I want to share with everyone, but can't until it's all proper and above board.

We will be stretched financially for a few years until Osh goes to school, but we spend money on holidays anyway so we won't have to now, as we will have our 'holiday home' as the site owners call them. Rhodri was very sniffy about that as he has a bit of a problem with the term 'holiday home' – it's a Welsh-speaking thing, I think. I am calling it our 'caravan of lurve' as Rhodri and I never argue when we are on holiday because, funnily enough, I don't have the three hundred things I normally have to think about swimming around in my head.

This house, beautiful though it is, is a trap, as when I am here I think about all the things I should be doing like washing and ironing and gardening, putting the bins out, painting doors and walls, so all this will be gone if I escape. I will be able to spend time, exclusively devoted to my children and my husband, on beaches and walking through fields and on hills, in the sunshine, in the rain and thinking about nothing but them and what a bloody brilliant thing life is. We will for ever have those memories, and no one can take them away from us.

February 13, Tuesday

I've been on the phone to a lovely man in the caravan park in Kilgetty. God, I would never have believed how difficult it is to get a place in a caravan park in Tenby. I made a few phone calls to sites to ask if I could put my own van there, but you have to buy a van off them to get on their sites, unless it is a new van, which we can't afford.

Everyone I called would say, 'Have you bought a van before?' Then they would make this noise like 'Ah, here we go again.' BUT I think we have found something that fits all criteria from a lovely caravan-site-owning man with a very bad cold: a second-hand van a few miles from the beach with an indoor swimming pool on site. It also has a club which we might avoid, but not if we run out of wine one night, PLUS Elis loves a game of bingo (well, me under the guise of Elis loving bingo).

Also, the man says we can let it out to friends and family

if we want. They have caravans which sleep eight, which means we can take our friends too. It's more expensive than I had envisaged, actually it is double the cost, but I am thinking, Bugger it, when Osh goes to school in a year or so I will be about £500 a month better off and I will just shop in cheaper places and not buy any clothes.

I do not in my heart of hearts even believe myself that those two things will happen, but I am saying it like a mantra because I will not be deterred. Would Richard Branson be where he is today without taking a few risks in life, I ask myself. Would *Tubular Bells* ever have seen the light of day or those aeroplanes, or that balloon – actually I think that balloon crashed, didn't it, so I won't think too much about that. So we which always means me, are arranging to go down there on Sunday if possible to have a look at the site and some caravans.

I went to Welsh class today and Janet the teacher said, 'Michelle, translate into Welsh "May I have a lift?"' so I said, 'Gaf i godiad?' and she nearly choked, and when I asked what the matter was she said, 'You just said, "May I have an erection?"': *Godiad* means erection in Welsh so Teri and I scribbled it down immediately in our vocabulary books and were giggling like two teenagers. 'Very useful for Valentine's Day tomorrow,' I said and we giggled even more and Janet said, 'No, don't write it down, as someone might report me to WLPAN,' (the people who run the course) but we said her secret was safe with us.

Went home and asked Rhodri how his *codiad* was and he was shocked that I said it, so shocked he got one which we made use of; now he owes me a further £3.333 (recurring).

February 14, Wednesday

Valentine's Day. I had a card from a secret admirer –

Rhodri has been writing that for the last ten years, I wonder if he realises I know it's him, I know his handwriting. We all ate Marks & Spencer's hand-decorated Valentine's chocolates for breakfast. I kept one for Kerry though, as she is also my Valentine for being so lovely.

Kerry came over as I was putting my make-up on without my wig. She is the only person other than Rhodri and Elis, and my sister once, who I allow to see me without my wig. I was about to put it back on and she said, 'Put it on Daisy,' and we put it on her and it was hilarious. We laughed so much we were crying, and Kerry said she had to go to the toilet because she was going to pee herself. I can't remember a time when I have laughed like that – it really is the best medicine.

Elis went to Alex's house after school and I picked him up about 7.30 with Osh in his pyjamas. Rhodri had been queuing outside the American Embassy for three hours to get a visa and didn't get back until nine. He was so cold in the queue he nearly cried. I said to Elis, 'Did you do anything for Valentine's Day in school?' and he said, 'No, Miss Smith gave everyone Valentine's cards except me.' I expressed my doubts over this. He continued, 'And some of the children in the class had Valentine's cards off each other and I didn't have any,' and just as I was thinking it was a bit grown-up for seven year olds to be exchanging Valentines, Elis said in a really sad voice, 'You know, Mum, just because I am a small person doesn't mean that I don't want to have a Valentine's card,' and my heart skipped a beat.

A bit later I was tucking him up in bed and I remembered that Osh had made a Valentine's card (as well as a biscuit which he opened and ate on the way home) and I said, 'Oh, you did have a Valentine's card. I forgot – it's in the car,' and he said, 'Who is it from?' I said, 'It's from Osh,' and he smiled and said, 'Was there any chocolate with it?' 'Oh yes, lots of chocolate,' I said, 'You can have it in the morning,' and he went to bed smiling.

Will have to raid the chocolate lips I bought Rhodri and put them in an envelope with the card for the morning because even small people need a bit of extra love on Valentine's Day.

February 15, Thursday

I'm a bit post-Valentine's Day hungover – teetotalling not going terribly well at the moment, but will not drink until I get to Ireland on Sunday. It would be rude, nay tantamount to a sin, not to drink in Ireland. Went for a long walk with Rhodri today across the coastal path in Llantwit Major; it was really lovely, very bracing, blowing all my cobwebs away. I just thought how great it will be to be able to go to the sea with the children. Children and coastal paths do not mix, especially with 300-foot drops and subsidence. Elis would have to be about twenty-seven before I would let him go there on his own.

Had a letter through today about my mammogram. It's on 26 March. I am glad to have it, but will now spend the next six weeks worrying about it – worrying about something I can't actually do anything about.

I still have a very slight discharge coming from my nipple, and whenever I search it in Google, which ever way I do it, it says it is not likely to be breast cancer but to get it checked out. Rhodri said, 'Don't worry about it. They're not worried about it in the hospital, so you don't need to be either.'

Before I had my diagnosis I wouldn't have worried, but I was told they were almost certain nothing was wrong and yet I *did* have breast cancer the first time. So it is inevitable that I will worry after what I have just gone through. I start thinking, What if the cancer does come back – what then?

Just snapped at Rhodri as it's eight o'clock and he's

letting Elis start an art project in his room when he should be sleeping. He said, 'What can I do about it?' I said, 'You're the adult, he's taking the piss out of you. You should have told him to get into bed.' Then he said, 'I can't do anything right,' and I said, 'In this case, no,' and he said, 'Piss off,' and I said, 'Piss off,' and I threw the first thing that came to hand at him; which was a brush. I wonder if my period is due (my usual explanation for my irrational behaviour). I am supposed to be keeping a record of it but I forgot. I think I might be pre-menstrual. Was hoping I would never have a period again, but hey ho, we'll see.

February 27, Tuesday

Haven't managed to get to my diary for a while as I was in Ireland for a week. I had forgotten about my diary, in fact, and about most other things too, like I have had cancer and chemotherapy. I was much more moderate in my behaviour while in the Emerald Isle than in previous years, but I still had a few drinks with my sister.

Then I spent most of the holiday beating myself up about this, but my sister says that as long as it is now and again, I should stop being so hard on myself. I have started to get anxiety attacks. Well, I'm not even sure what they are, but it's that feeling of dread, that something bad is going to happen, and you have a flutter in your chest, not palpitations exactly, but a sensation like that. I am wondering what this is all about. There is a niggling feeling about the mammogram and until I have it and someone tells me everything is OK, I won't rest easy.

I'm still really excited about the caravan and spent some of the time in Ireland researching sites and caravan costs, the one wevisited was a apossibility but I'd prefer something closer to the sea. I do feel slightly middle-aged doing all this but this really is going to be a facet of my life that I think will bring me great pleasure. I so love being in Pembrokeshire by the sea, it's so invigorating, and when Rhodri comes too I can go for walks on the beach as we do when we are on holidays; it really does have a spiritual dimension to it. I said to Rhodri that I was a little apprehensive about buying a caravan before my mammogram, as if it was bad news we might have committed ourselves to something we couldn't afford. And he sat by me and put his arm around me and said that I can't live my life thinking the worst will happen, and that I have to live my life thinking this is not going to be a problem and I said but what if it was, and he said that, if that happened – which it wasn't going to – we would cross that bridge when we came to it.

I am feeling anxious writing this now. Maybe after the mammogram it will get easier; if not, I'm straight back to Deborah for some counselling. I'm also thinking about going back to work, which I do want to do, but I think it is going to be a bit overwhelming, and then I think this is ridiculous because I am worrying about something that is going to happen in June and I haven't even had my radiotherapy yet.

In my head I've done it and that's part of the problem, if it is a problem, of being so positive about everything because you forget you are ill, and then I think, Shit I've still got to have radiotherapy. I just don't think it can be as bad as chemo or looking after your children for a week at half-term.

We had a lovely time in Ireland, although we managed to miss the flight because of a crash on the motorway. It was very serious and they closed the motorway; I thought they usually only do that when someone has been killed and was not going to get stressed about us missing the plane when someone could have lost their life.

This resolve lasted about five minutes. I called Ryanair and they said they could get us on a flight going to Dublin –

we were originally going to Shannon – but that was fine and the car hire company was at both airports so no problem there, and it would cost £50.

When we got there, we were told it would cost £50 EACH to change – £200 – which was more than the original flights. We could have had a round-the-world trip for the cost of those flights and it stinks because no one would have taken those seats at an hour's notice. So I was Outraged From Cardiff and asked for Ryanair's details to write them a letter, which I have done now, asking for £150 back.

We will see but Aidan says I haven't got a hope in hell of getting it back, although we did have mitigating circumstances.

Anyway, we were in the lift going to Departures and there was a woman in the lift who must have thought I was mad. I was fuming and saying to Rhodri, 'Well, it just makes me so fucking angry,' and he was saying, 'Just shut your fucking mouth. I paid the money, stop going on about it,' and I said, 'It has spoiled my fucking holiday,' and Elis piped up, 'Now, guys, there's no point swearing about it.' That told us, it really was like the Haribo advert. Travelling makes me even more irritable than I normally am.

The children got on so well on holiday. I hardly spoke to Elis for six days as he and Diarmuid were so happy together. Fintan is a year older than Osh, and they were the greatest of pals.

Rhodri and Aidan went walking a few times, and Rhodri got a tick on him which I had to remove with tweezers and pour tea-tree oil on. Sarah had said to be careful of ticks and he had laughed, then came home and there was one half-burrowed into his skin – dead. There must be something in Rhodri's skin to repel Irish ticks. It probably gave up after the first layer (hope Rhodri never reads this).

It was Rhodri's birthday two days ago. He is now thirty-six years old, still a pup really. We stayed in and I cooked us steaks and bought him a speaker for his Ipod and the boys (very generous things that they are) bought him a rucksack.

Rhodri and I are off to Portmeirion tomorrow, such is our jet-set life. I had to get it in before radiotherapy as it is for three nights and I won't be able to go afterwards as I have to go before the end of March. So just as I've unpacked, ironed and put away from Ireland, I need to start again. Don't know how pop stars manage but they have 'people' to do things for them, no doubt.

Osh is going up to the farm tonight and Julia is picking Elis up from school tomorrow; Joanne is taking him on Friday. I hope I am able to repay all these favours one day and that people aren't getting fed up with me. I'm also hoping radiotherapy will be easy as I have not really planned otherwise and Rhodri is away for most of March filming Al Bowlly and possibly also has to go to America. Oh, it's a tough life being a TV director, don't you know. He says he doesn't want to go and leave us, but if I had the opportunity to go to New York, stay in a nice hotel without two children and a moaning wife, I think I might just be looking forward to it a little bit, even if it is work.

Elis told me last night that he is singing in the school concert on Thursday, when Rhodri and I will be on our way to Portmeirion. I say we won't be here, and if he had told us earlier we might have been able to come. He said he forgot to tell us and was sobbing in bed. So I had to promise him two packs of football cards, which he is obsessed with, because I knew he was going to be great singing, even if we weren't there to see him. He said, 'Where are you going?' and I said, 'I told you, we're going to Portmeirion where we went for our honeymoon.' Whenever you mention honeymoon, he says, 'That's zexy.' He always says sexy with a 'z' for some reason, despite my correcting him. So I said, 'We are going to Portmeirion where we had our sexy honeymoon,' and he said, 'Have you ever had zex with

234

Rhodri?' and I said, 'Yes I have.' He said, 'You don't even know what zex is,' and I said, 'Yes, I do, it's when Daddy puts his pee pee in Mummy's foo foo and you have a baby.'

'Yes, that's right,' he said, 'so you and Rhodri have had zex twice, once for me and once for Osian.' I didn't elaborate.

I'm getting very hot at nights and am wondering if I'm having hot flushes and starting the menopause. Although I still don't know when my period is due. Actually, I just looked back through my diary and think it was 17 January, but that seems a long time ago – well, it was a long time ago, or it could be that the duvets in Ireland were very warm. I've also been really hot at night back home. If they are flushes then they are fine, but I can't believe they are, as every woman I know who has had them says they are pretty unbearable. So we shall see. At least I will save myself a fortune in jumpers.

My hair is growing back with a vengeance, so much so that I'm not wearing my little black hat at night. I used to think, God, I can't go out with grey hair, now I don't think it will bother me. I just want my hair back. I actually shampooed and conditioned it in the bath yesterday for the first time since I shaved it all off. Sarah had said, 'You'd better start looking after that,' and she is right. It did feel really soft. I now have some hair to run my fingers through but it is still very short and looks post-chemo as opposed to elfin Mia Farrow. I read an article with the lovely Kylie and she said she didn't know whether to keep her hair Mia Farrow-like and I thought, Kylie, you'd look fab wearing a binliner and no hair.

I feel I have to lose at least a stone before I can go commando on the hair front because there are many words to describe me and elfin is not one of them. Chubby chops and short hair have never been a great look, methinks.

When I was in Ireland and Diarmuid and Elis were tormenting Osian and I was just out of the shower in my bra and knickers with no wig on (I keep forgetting to put my wig on in the house as my hair is growing back a bit), so I went into the bedroom to tell them off and they were hysterical the pair of them, lying on the floor rolling about laughing because I looked so ridiculous in my bra and knickers with my 'bold head' as Elis calls it.

'See, Diarmuid?' Elis said. 'That's why my mother wears a wig,' and I couldn't tell them off, I was laughing so much because I did look ridiculous. Children are great levellers.

February 28, Wednesday

After a courageous battle with illness over many years, 'Fishy' finally lost his fight for life. Cleaning the fish along with washing my wig, emailing caravan parks and doing my Welsh homework was on my Things To Do list. By the time I got to poor old Fishy he was floating on the surface of the tank, never to be revived. I say this because I have caught him floating a few times before and have managed to revive him.

Apart from a growth on his head, he did not like water that was remotely dirty, and when we got back from Ireland it was a little murky. It all came too late. I fished him out immediately (no pun intended) and put him in another bowl, but he was lying there all gold and shiny-looking for all the world as if he were alive, except he was floating on his side. I poked him and tried to get him upright, but no amount of rebalancing or swishing about in clean water was going to revive him. He was as dead as they come.

I felt like shit about it because I should have cleaned him out sooner. I cleaned the tank immediately so that 'Rods' didn't go the same way. In the middle of it all the phone rang and it was my mother. I told her what had happened, and that I was upset and she said, 'Tell Elis you'll get another.'

I said, 'I don't want another, they're a pain. I'm the only one who ever takes any notice of them and cleans them, and I feel guilty when they die.' She was VERY sympathetic and said she knew exactly how I felt as Emily had them when she was younger and they were always dying, and Mum was always replacing them and cleaning the bloody tank out. We bonded hugely over the responsibility that goes with a goldfish that every child has to have but none of them ever look after. I picked Elis up from school and was dreading telling him, because the last time one of his fish died, although he hadn't looked at them for years and I thought he wasn't going to be too upset by it and had already flushed it down the toilet, he was hysterical and traumatised then wanted to see him – so I had to say I had buried him in the garden. So we got in the car and I said, 'Elis, I have some very sad news for you. Your fish has died.' His bottom lip went for all of two seconds and he said, 'We can get another one.' Then he said, 'Which one?' and I said, 'The one with the orange thing on his head,' and he said, 'Oh, maybe we can get one that looks exactly the same, we'll just keep replacing him.'

Bloody hell, there he goes again, I thought. Something dies, just get another one. Like men and wives: just get a smarter, prettier, thinner version. Can't imagine Rhodri would go out and get a bald, size-fourteen-to-sixteen wife the next time round.

So as I was pulling away in the car Elis said, 'I knew he was going to die today.' I stopped the car and was a bit spooked by this, and I said, 'How?'

'Because the water looked a bit dirty,' he said.

'Oh, don't say that, I feel really bad now,' I said and he replied, 'You don't have to feel bad about it, Mum, it's not your fault. I'm the one who is supposed to be looking after him. I'm the fish killer.'

I said that he wasn't and that the fish was just ill and

these things happen. I did feel very guilty though, until I was in Tescos with him buying Rhodri an anniversary card and I told him he couldn't have something and he said, 'At least I'm not a fish killer.' Bastards, they have the knack of hitting you right where it hurts.

We went home and it turns out that Fishy is in fact Rods, although I was sure that wasn't the case. However, Rhodri and I were instructed by Elis to gather round and say a prayer. Elis said he didn't know what to say and asked me to say a few words and he told Rhodri off for not putting his hands together properly. So I thanked God for Rod's life and letting us be a part of it and asked Him to look after him in heaven.

Elis was very pleased with this. I said I would bury him in the garden but Elis said it might be better if we put him in a bowl in the garden, so that way we could see him every day. Ah, if only life were as simple as that. I did, of course, bury him in the garden – just like the last time our fish died.

March 1, Thursday

Hapus Dydd Dewi Sant. It is St David's Day today, but more importantly, it is our fifth wedding anniversary and Rhodri is taking me to Portmeirion where we spent our honeymoon all those years ago. Elis and Osh are going to their rural retreat – my parents' farm – and my lovely sisters are taking Elis up and down to Cardiff to school. God bless them! My favours must surely be running out, but when 'project vantastic' as I am now calling my caravan hunt comes off the ground and when my eight-berth 'holiday home' is up and running (except I am not allowed to call it that because of the Welsh Nationalist thing), I can let them holiday there and return all the hundreds of favours they have done for me during my illness. I do know in my heart of hearts that they do not need repaying and if there was

238

ever anything wrong with them, I would gladly do the same.

Elis was at the breakfast table this morning and I said, 'It's our wedding anniversary today, and we've been married for five years. You were two when we were married.'

He paused mid-Cheerios and did a double take. 'Well, who did you get the zex with?' he demanded.

'Well, Rhodri, of course,' I said.

'What, you don't have to be married to have zex?'

'No.'

'Oooh,' he said as if I had just told him the most interesting fact he had ever heard. I should have told him that yes, you did have to be married, then he would wait until his thirties before he popped his cherry.

Rhodri is Outraged From Cardiff because Elis comes home full of Bible stories – which I think are a very good grounding for morality and, to be honest, what did he expect, sending him to a traditional Welsh-language school? Although I'm not impressed that he said he learnt that Eve was naughty in the Garden of Eden, possibly setting the bedrock for a life of thinking women are the bad ones. Hey ho. But Rhodri and Elis have some very interesting conversations about the origins of life, as Rhodri is a firm non-believer and Elis is a firm Christian, although Rhodri said that I cannot call a seven year old a Christian because he doesn't know what it is to be a Christian. Based on that logic, I guess I shouldn't call him a football supporter either, because surely he doesn't know what that is at seven either!

Rhodri and Elis were discussing how life started and whether God created the earth in seven days. Rhodri told Elis this wasn't true: earth was created by the Big Bang which, according to Elis, was created by God. I love it – but I never get involved.

Arrived in Portmeirion about four. This is really one of

239

the most beautiful places in the world. I defy anyone to say otherwise. The view from our room over the estuary is magnificent. It is so peaceful here and the light changes by the minute.

March 2, Friday

We ate a five-course meal last night which was superb. Rhodri had a suit on with a black polo-neck jumper and looked very handsome, although he had brown socks on which were a bit of a no-no. Portmeirion is where they filmed *The Prisoner* and Rhodri really did look like Patrick McGoohan. I thought, God, I bet they think we are those *Prisoner* people who come here. Last time we were here there was a group of them and they dressed up in *Prisoner* outfits – fun, or a bit weird, I haven't decided yet. I could hardly walk by the end of the meal and by ten o'clock was sleeping like a baby. I was so hot all night, I was sweating and I thought I was definitely menopausal but Rhodri woke up and said, 'God, it's boiling in here,' and opened a window. So unless Rhodri is also menopausal then I can't be sure if the chemotherapy has pushed me over the menopausal edge.

Either way, there is no sign of a period, much to Rhodri's delight, as we have been at it like rabbits. This is married-couple speak for 'we've done it twice in two days'. We only have one condom left as I happened to have some in a toiletry bag from ages ago and Rhodri only brought one as he thought that was all the sex he would be getting.

'I view sex like I view Cardiff City,' he said. 'I never expect them to win and if they do, then it's a bonus.' I laughed.

I progressed 'project vantastic' a bit more. I rang one of the holiday parks and told the lady my budget and asked her what she could do for that. She said she could get me something for that amount but it would be a basic caravan. She named the two models I've been looking at anyway. We are going down next Sunday to have another look – ooh, it is so exciting. I keep thinking it's such a middle-aged thing to do, but then I think, God, I *am* middle-aged.

In Ireland I read an article about a woman who died of radiation poisoning from radiotherapy, but she had had her radiotherapy thirty-four years ago for breast cancer. Her husband said he wasn't bitter about it because they had given her thirty-four years of life.

I thought, Bloody hell, if I get thirty-four years of life after this I will be ecstatic! In the beginning I used to think, Give me five years, then give me ten. Then I think, No, give me thirty-four or more.

Caravan park owners give you a time limit for keeping your caravan on their site; the one I'm interested in is fifteen years. I will be fifty-five by then and I will be very, very happy to get there. Turning forty means nothing. I wonder why anyone who has had cancer gives a toss about how old they are. As each year passes you've notched up another year in spite of it; you've stuck two fingers up to cancer and you've got on with your life.

I am looking out of the window as I write, the light is hitting the mountains and it looks more like a painting. I feel truly at rest and at peace, with nothing to do, nowhere to go, just sitting looking through the window at the herons fishing and the geese flying overhead. I've got the window wide open, it's so warm. I can see why poets and writers and artists want to live here. It is inspirational – but bloody cold in winter, I bet.

We went for a walk this morning and a robin followed us all over the place. When we sat down it was inches away from my shoulder and it kept trying to sit on Rhodri; it was amazing, I took photos of it and it wasn't put off by the flash. It is probably paid by Portmeirion to make the guests feel special and at one with nature, which we do.

There was a rainbow over the estuary yesterday evening right after we had our first shag. It's a sign of brighter things to come. Maybe Cardiff will go up to the Premiership this season.

March 4, Sunday

Left lovely Portmeirion for another few years. The next time we go we'll take the children, although we said that the last time, and I thought by the time our tenth anniversary comes along, Osh will be eight and Elis will be twelve. It seems another lifetime away, although Elis has teenage tendencies already so I'm not sure what he will be like when he actually is a teenager.

We stopped off at Rhodri's parents on the way back for lunch. We haven't seen them since Christmas. Rhodri's mother asked me about my treatment and I had forgotten about it. I thought, Shit, yes, I'm having radiotherapy on Thursday and it has completely gone out of my mind! I've mentally ticked it off as I think it will be OK, like Helen the breast nurse said when she was going through everything: 'After chemotherapy, radiotherapy is a walk in the park,' so I am hoping that I will be walking in the park for the next month.

I have made no arrangements for the children and fully expect to take myself to and from it, as Rhodri is away for most of this month. So, basically, I'm on my own. I know my mother will step in if I need her but Elis has to go to school, so I have to stay here.

Arrived at the farm around 6.30 p.m. to pick the children up. I gave them the presents I had bought them. Lloyd and Elis had footballs – a big mistake, as try telling a four year old and a seven year old not to kick them around the house, but all the gifts went down well.

I have won a television in the school raffle, hurrah! I

can't believe it, I have never won anything in my life before and I will need a television for 'project vantastic' when it comes to fruition. I said to Rhodri that maybe I should give it back to the school and he said, 'For Christ's sake, Shelley, don't be a martyr all your life. You won the television, take the television.' So I did.

March 5, Monday

I have been trying to do Welsh, but the house is in chaos so it's a bit difficult. I will definitely sit the exam but may not be able to keep up if my appointments clash with the lessons this month. Either way, I am continuing with it as I *will* speak it, and, if I can get the hang of mutations, then I can conquer anything.

Rhodri and I have started doing Weight Watchers together. We don't do the classes, we just do it at home. I have bought Weight Watchers bathroom scales for us and Rhodri and I are very excited about it. Until I bought them I would not have any scales in the house in case I became obsessed with weighing myself. However, what this means is that I never know if I am putting on weight, so now I do need to monitor myself. I want to make sure when I whip my wig off for all the world to see that I'm not looking like a balding Billy Bunter.

Elis said, 'Your hair is growing back really nicely, Mum,' and I thought what a lovely thing it was to say, but then he added, 'But it's grey so that must mean you are really old.' It is mainly grey and I've only just hit forty. My grandmother was grey from a very young age so I guess I take after her – along with the martyrdom element to my personality, which I also share with her.

March 6, Tuesday

Bugger, bugger, bugger. The woman at the caravan park who said she could sort me out a nice van for my budget now tells me she can't. I cannot believe how complicated this caravan malarkey is. I have spent three hours on the internet and ringing caravan sites trying to arrange some appointments for Sunday, as Rhodri isn't around after that for a month, so if we don't see anything suitable on Sunday it will be ages before we can get anything sorted.

The weather at the moment is glorious and I keep thinking we could be down at our caravan this weekend – if we could get one. After all my phone calls I've found three possibilities in a beautiful area where we went on holiday a few years ago, so if any of them is any good we will be taking it there and then. Except I haven't actually got the money yet, so will have to take my credit card.

Joanne and Mum did their Kim and Aggie bit and came down and rescued me from the house, which was threatening to consume me with clothes and mess. Yesterday afternoon I fell asleep in the chair and my mother rang and I said I was tired, and she said, 'Yes, you have suffered an emotional trauma,' (not the attempt to do the housework but the cancer). Usually I dismiss such statements but it's difficult to remember that it is a big bloody emotional trauma.

You concentrate on all the physical elements of your illness and of course you know that it is upsetting and distressing, but it *is* an emotional trauma and that in itself is exhausting.

Alison K rang and asked me how I was and I said I was tired but I couldn't remember if this is how tired I felt before all of this, as I was always tired, and that was because I had two small children and a husband who was never around. She said, 'If it's any consolation, Neil and I are permanently exhausted.' I think that's just a parent's lot in life, when you have small children.

I definitely think I have menopausal symptoms. I have been reading on the internet that chemotherapy can cause the menopause but can also cause menopausal symptoms, thus having the symptoms without having the menopause, but in my age bracket there is an 80 per cent chance that I will actually have the menopause. I definitely have the hot flushes, although they are nothing I can't handle.

The other major thing is that my periods have stopped (hurrah) and also I keep getting waves of anxiety washing over me, a bit like when you have to stand up and give a presentation which you don't want to do but know you have to. I couldn't understand what the anxiety was really about, but it's something that happens when you have the menopause apparently. Now I know that, I don't feel so bad, as I was thinking there was something else wrong with me.

I told Rhodri this, as I've been asking myself what I'm so anxious about all the time. Then I proceeded to go through the list of other conditions associated with the menopause and asked him if he'd noticed them in me, like aggressiveness, irritability, anger, headaches, or mood swings. By the end of reading the list he was laughing in a mildly hysterical way as he says (yet again) he's not going to know the difference between the pre- and post-menopausal me.

Apparently there is a test you can take which tells you if you are menopausal, although you are only finally declared menopausal after six months without periods. Sage tea is good for hot flushes. I have bought the tea but have yet to drink any. Just owning it makes me feel better already.

March 7, Wednesday

I have been gardening today and my back feels as if

someone has jumped on it. The good news is that after two years of traipsing up and down the garden with our compostable waste, I can actually use it. I have real compost; it actually works! It is a very satisfying, self-righteous feeling to think that my plant pots are filled with all the stuff that we have thrown out and which would have otherwise ended up in landfill. Me and Al Gore will single-handedly be saving the planet.

Had lunch with Manon today in the Japanese – very nice and we had a glass of wine and felt very naughty. Manon has left the BBC and has started doing 'The House of Colour'. She looks at all the colours that suit you, depending on your own colouring. She offered to do mine but I was a bit worried that she might tell me that black is not my colour, as it tends to make me look a bit washed-out but I have an entire wardrobe full of black as it's very slimming. I must do lunch more often. When I leave the house I really enjoy it but I convince myself I have to do all these jobs which will still be here when I get back.

Radiotherapy tomorrow. Rhodri at the eleventh hour says do I want him to come with me and I say yes as I don't know what it will be like. I am sure it will be fine, but it would be good to have someone there. I hope to God they don't nuke the wrong bit of me.

March 8, Thursday

I thought radiotherapy might be like that scene in one of the James Bond movies when Sean Connery, I think, is lying on a bed; there's a laser beam slicing through the metal plate he is lying on and it's about to cut him in half – starting with his lovely Scottish manhood. Luckily, he escapes somehow or other. So I thought I would lie there and an enormous laser beam would come out of a machine and be very noisy and zap the relevant tattooed place on my breast . It wasn't anything like that.

Before you go in, the nurse goes through the list of possible side-effects like being tired and having sore skin. You have to use Simple soap or Dove, nothing perfumed and no deodorant. I only use Crystal deodorant now as I know there is aluminium in ordinary deodorants. Aluminium is not good for you and there is talk that there could be a link with it and breast cancer, so I stopped using it, ironically about a month before I got my diagnosis. Apparently, as regards being tired, like chemo it is cumulative, but I said I hadn't made any provisions for anyone to look after me or my children. The nurse told me that if I am going to be tired it will be in a few weeks, the soreness the same, but some people don't feel tired at all, and anyway it is nothing like the chemotherapy tiredness. I will be able to carry on with what I normally do, I'll just be a bit tired.

So that was all very reassuring. I was a bit worried it might be like an enclosed MRI machine, which I had a scan in once, and it's bloody awful if you are claustrophobic like me. She said, no, it was not like that.

The machine is very high-tech, a *Star-Trek*-type thing which is a bit daunting but also reassuring as it looks like it can do the business. So you lie there and they line up your tattoos with something and there are two, sometimes three people, all checking and double checking your alignment with the machine. They leave the room (so they don't get zapped) then it makes this humming noise, then it stops and they come back in, realign the machine and approach the tumour from a different angle, then that's it. All very painless and straightforward really, so I am very glad about it all. When I came out after about five minutes, Rhodri said, 'Oh that's it, is it?' So I don't have to worry about driving back and forth in future.

The waiting room is in a different part of the hospital

and the people look less sick and have more hair, so it's not as depressing as the chemo side. All in all, I feel as if I am progressing now to better health.

March 9, Friday

I have decided that I am going to drop Welsh for the rest of the year. After struggling with those bloody treiglads and finally having some understanding as to why they mutate, I don't think realistically I can carry on for the next four weeks. A lot of my appointments are near to twelve o'clock, they have already juggled them about to fit in with a school day and I know how difficult it is to get on the radiotherapy machines, so I could not possibly ask them to fit the appointments around my Welsh class as well, especially seeing that I will also miss another week in May, when we go on holiday.

I will do my exam for the first half of the Welsh course and pick it up again in September, so at least I would have achieved something; I am determined to carry on with it as I really feel that I am getting somewhere.

In a way it is a bit of a relief. It's odd having gone through chemotherapy, which is by far the worst bit, and managing to keep up with the classes. For some reason it seems all a bit too much to do at the moment. When Rhodri isn't here I have to get the children up and off to school, then come back, have a tidy up, then off to radiotherapy, where you can wait for over an hour just to get seen sometimes. It's just very time-consuming, and then to have to think about going to Welsh and doing two hours' work and then having to come back and get the children and do the tea and put them to bed by myself, it's bloody hard work.

I think I might be trying to convince myself here a bit too. I've come this far and I shouldn't be so hard on myself, because I've kept going through some very difficult times and it's not lost and I can still do some studying over the summer. I will make a determined effort to speak it with Rhodri and Elis and Osh so that I'm using it.

March 10, Saturday

Rhodri took Elis and Jay to the footie and I utilised the opportunity to take Osh on a shopping trip for more stuff for 'project vantastic'. The attic will be groaning under the weight of it all before long. I am crossing items off my 'things to buy' list; all I need is a caravan to put them all in. We are going to Tenby tomorrow to have a look at three sites and I hope that we will be able to find something that's right for us. Now that the nights are lighter and the weather isn't as depressing as it has been all winter, I want to be down there living my 'holiday home' dream. I did once say that I would never go on holiday in a caravan and laughed at the whole scene; that was before I had children and realised that you cannot afford to go abroad more than once a year, and that is usually on a credit card in our case, that children don't give a toss about the weather or the number of stars your hotel has, they want a bucket and spade, a football, a beach, an ice cream and a pool and they are like little pigs in muck.

I realised this the first time we went to Tenby on holiday. We spent three years taking Elis to beautiful unspoilt islands and they were lovely, but we could go out of season when there were few people around. Suddenly school starts and you are on this hamster treadmill with everyone else; you have to go at the hottest time of the year (and I am not good in the sun) and pay astronomical prices, and when you get there it's full of people.

The truth is, no matter what the weather, Elis is on the beach and as happy there in our little West Wales cottage as if we had just spent two thousand pounds on a five-star chalet. So we started holidaying there and haven't stopped, really. Every time I go there I remember the first holiday we ever had as a family in a cottage near the beach. Elis was three months old and I looked in the visitor book last year, when we went just before I had my diagnosis, and I had written that he had us up at five o'clock every morning. I remember taking him along the sea-front in his pushchair without a living soul around, and Rhodri and I taking shifts to be with him because he was so exhausting. We didn't have a bloody clue about getting him off to sleep or into a routine. It's as if that place has grown up with us as parents and with our children. When I come over the hill and see the town and the sea I always make a little 'ah' sound. It's like seeing an old friend whom you really love and that's why I want my caravan in Tenby. I feel at peace there.

March 11, Sunday

We have found a site and a caravan – hurrah, hurrah, hurrah! I can't believe it. We went around the three sites we had arranged to see. The first one would be a bit like Magaluf in the summer, it was so big; the second one was nice but basically a collection of static caravans in a field and not much else, and the third one was tiny and a bit run down, and I just couldn't see us there, really.

So we passed a caravan site we stayed on two years ago which is by a church that had a banner on it saying, *Miracles Can Happen* and I thought, Well, not today they haven't. The site is a five-star one, with swimming pool and a club (Elis still talks about the bingo games we had there, and that was two years ago), and a gym and sauna and two play parks, and also a lovely garden centre next door with a really nice café, and the station is right behind the camp.

Rhodri said, 'Have you tried there?' I said, 'Yes, I have,

and they emailed back and said they didn't have any, plus we couldn't afford it.' So he said, 'Well, just go in and ask.' I went in and said we'd stayed there a few years ago and asked if they had any caravans for sale, and they did. I couldn't believe it.

They showed us one which was not really suitable and the man said, 'If you come back in a few hours, there's another one which will be empty and I'll show you that.' So we had lunch and went to the beach and came back; he showed it to us and it was perfect. It's a few years old and has the obligatory clashing carpets and upholstery, and it's not squeaky clean new, but it is good inside and in a nice spot with a bit of green behind it. The site is clean and tidy, and the site owners are quite strict. They want to know who is in the caravans so that families feel they can let their children go to the park on their own without worrying. There is a barrier entry to the site, so you can't just drive onto it like the other three we went to see. So we sat down with them and they went through all the costs; we said we'd take all the details home with us and look at our finances. So we drove back and worked it all out, and if the truth be told it is a lot of money to pay in fees. We can't really afford it, but, bugger it, we're having it anyway. The children would have grown up and left home by the time we can actually afford anything, so if we don't do it now, we never will. I want to be there in Tenby with my children who drive me mad sometimes, but they might as well be driving me mad in Tenby as at home in Cardiff.

March 12, Monday

'Project vantastic' has come to fruition, and we are now the proud owners of a Willerby Westmorland caravan. The deal is done, I've paid the deposit and as soon as the money comes through – hopefully this week – it is ours. My treatment finishes on 4th April, which is the first week of the Easter holidays, so it means that we can be down there for the rest of the holidays. I say 'we', but Rhodri will be working for some of the time. However, I can take the children as long as the radiotherapy hasn't zapped me, and maybe my mother or Joanne will come to help me get it all set up. It is so exciting. I will stop buying clothes, I will shop more cheaply, and I will limit my eBay purchases to absolute essentials only. I will be a new, less materialistic, beach-combing, caravan-owning, serene, in-touch-with-nature-and-my-children, mother. Ah!

March 19, Monday

God knows what I have been doing this week but I never seem to have a minute to myself. Having radiotherapy is a bit like having a job suddenly. I know it's not an eight-hour day, but I've gone from doing nothing for long periods of time to suddenly having to be somewhere every day on time. How the hell I am going to do my real job, and all the hundred other things I also do, is beyond me. I keep thinking. How did I manage to fit all this in before? I know there is a tendency to fill the time with the amount of work you have to do, but I forget that I basically ran around like a blue-arsed fly, completely stressed out all the time, never sitting down until about ten o'clock at night, not going to bed until about twelve. God, no wonder I drank alcohol.

It is so easy to see, when you can sit back and think, that this is a stressful life, yet thousands of women do it every day, all of the time. I know that men, well, some of them, do their bit and I know Rhodri genuinely believes he does half of what needs doing in this house, but he doesn't and if I say that to him he goes mad. He doesn't see all the hundreds of little jobs that he has NEVER had to do. He has never cleaned either the toilet or the bathroom – he wouldn't know where to start. He has never washed a floor, he has never sewed any of Elis's clothes, he doesn't iron, he has never done any of the painting in this house. I know he would do them IF I ASKED. That is what infuriates me about men. They say, 'All you have to do is ask,' and you think, If I had to be asked for every single thing I did in this house, nothing would get done.

I DON'T WANT TO HAVE TO ASK. I want him to see that something needs doing, and do it, like I do, not complain about it, not whine to me that he has had to fill the dishwasher three times. All I do for most of the week is fill and empty the insatiable gaping hole that is the dishwasher. Men never fail to amaze me. Rhodri has a very responsible job – he is a director who works on productions where sometimes there are hundreds of people to orchestrate and position, and he works with set designers and lighting directors and cameramen and orchestras and singers and a whole team of support people, to produce hours, sometimes, of television – and I cannot for one minute imagine him sitting there and staring into space until someone asks him to do something.

Oh no, because that is the world of work which is his domain and he is the one who is doing the asking there, he is the one who takes control and gets people motivated and works it all out because work is what is really important, and anything that *isn't* work is unimportant and he really doesn't want to do it. It's not just Rhodri, it is most men who are like that.

The older I have become, the more I realise that men and women are never going to get it right. Along with many of my female friends, and we are all educated women with good jobs, we feel that our families, our children, are central to our existence.

I'm not saying that Elis and Osh are not central to Rhodri's existence, because they are; it is just that for us, children are the number one thing and everything else orbits around them. We would give up our careers tomorrow if we thought that it affected our children adversely, but men are defined by their work in a way that we don't feel we have to be.

I just think I am forty, a mother of two children, I don't feel that I have anything to prove to anyone. It's not having had cancer, although that just serves to strengthen it, it is because for me being a mother is the most fundamental part of my existence. I grew two human beings inside my womb and I have to look after them, and although I consider myself to be a feminist, in many ways having those children has re-shaped my existence. It's not as if I'm one of these middle-class, breastfeeding-up-to-the-age-of-four earth mothers. I'm not like that, that's just the way it is for me.

God, I'm not sure where this rant is coming from, other than this weekend I was sick and tired of tidying up because tidying up with children in the house is like trying to hit a moving target, it's virtually impossible. I asked Rhodri if he would tidy Elis's bedroom and he said, 'You could ask me in a proper voice,' and I said, 'That was my proper voice.' OK, it was a little on the terse side, but if I had a pound for every time I have cleaned that room, I would be living in the Bahamas by now.

I said, 'I'm just sick of tidying this bloody house,' and Rhodri said, 'I have filled the dishwasher three times today.'

'That's what I have to do every day of the bloody week,' I said crossly, 'but it is so dull and monotonous that I cannot bring myself to tell you about it, unlike you, who thinks that you are a martyr doing the things I do every bloody, boring day of my life.'

God, I desperately need a job but, if I have a job, will it all descend into chaos and be too stressful? Will I be able to cope with it all? What I need is a wife, just like me, well actually without the nagging bit, to look after me.

My menopausal symptoms continue. I haven't seen

Rosie for a few weeks, with one thing and another, but saw her today and she said radiotherapy can give you flushes like that because it's heating up your body. I also have the night sweats where you go to bed perfectly normal and wake up in a ball of perspiration. Fortunately my sleep doesn't seem to be affected by it. I just have a drink of water and kick the blankets off and go back to sleep. I do think that I am very irritable and moody, especially with Rhodri and Elis. Elis has been driving me mad. I went to *Lord of the Dance* on Saturday, which was absolutely fab and I really did want to rip the male dancers' shirts off and have sex with them – thus proving that the sex drive can always come back when you want it to. My Auntie Janet came with me, as did my mother and my sister.

Janet has three boys who have grown up now, and she said that with her eldest she always felt that she had to have the last word because he would never let it drop, and I said I was the same with Elis. She said you have to ignore it and turn your back on them and walk away, otherwise you will be at loggerheads for years and she is right.

Had a cheque through for the caravan, but it is in both our names. We have never had a joint account – a very shrewd move on Rhodri's part, who no doubt picked up very early on that I am a spendaholic – and so we now have to wait for a cheque in just my name, so this has delayed us. I'm hoping though, that the caravan-selling man, Bob, will let us go there on Friday without the money in the account. I'll call tomorrow and ask in my loveliest voice.

Kate came over on Friday with MARK, yes, her man. He is very nice and she seems very relaxed in his company. Kate called in for a drink and ended up staying for dinner – I am trying to perfect Coq au Vin. I cooked it once for my mother, Sarah and Aidan and they have made jokes about it ever since (heathens). So Kate and Mark had some food and I kept topping up my and Kate's wine glass and was quite drunk by the end. Mark kept saying to Kate, 'We should go, we have to get up early in the morning,' and Kate kept saying, 'I'll have a drop more, Shelley,' and Rhodri said that Mark could see his leg-over slipping away with every glass of wine Kate had!

Radiotherapy is fine, no problems at all, although the waiting is a bit of a pain. They kept me waiting for two hours one day because someone had forgotten to tell me that I needed to report to reception, which I had been told *not* to do the day before, by someone else. So I was there for an hour watching everyone go in before I mentioned it, and then I was annoyed that they had seen me there for an hour and not said anything. There was another woman there and the same thing happened to her as well. We were saying to each other that they could see us there, etcetera and I said to her, 'I don't know why I'm complaining, I've got nothing else to do,' and she said, 'No, I haven't either.'

I did feel unreasonably pissed off for being kept waiting when actually they are saving my life, which I should perhaps concentrate on, rather than thinking this is an inconvenient thing I have to do every day. I am forgetting that this increases my chances of that cancer NOT coming back by 20 per cent, so I should remember that when I am in the waiting room. I will take my Ipod and try to rescue the little Welsh I have left in my deteriorating brain for my exam, and will not notice the time then.

So I will be going forward this week as the new, less shouty mummy and the less complaining patient. I'm hoping this sits well with the menopausal-hot-flushing, moody, irritable me. It is just a state of mind, it is just a state of mind. I have already killed a spider this morning and I'm now thinking this is bad karma. I must do something to make amends somewhere to re-order the universe, if indeed this is possible now.

March 20, Tuesday

The self-help books by the side of my bed are about two foot high and covered in dust. I put them there so I can dip into them before I go to sleep. I have yet to pick up a novel and read one, which was part of my great master plan, as I feel that it would involve too much engagement and cerebral effort on my part. So they remain on the beautiful bookshelves we have had put up, reflecting to the world our intelligence and good taste, but they too are gathering dust.

My true bedside friends at this moment are *Hello* magazine (especially two issues on Liz Hurley's wedding) and the Argos catalogue – for essential caravan purchases – and these alone have overtaken my need for self-help reading.

I actually look upon *Hello* and the Argos catalogue as a form of self-help in their own right – escapism and retail therapy. They should be on prescription. There was a time in between treatments post-chemo when I had my meltdown of sorts, when my self-help books were a much-needed crutch, but now they have come to represent a stage in my illness that I am not sure I want to go back to. Not yet, at least.

Here they are: *Cancer Positive, Say Fuck Off to Cancer* (actually *We Can Say No To Cancer*), *The Bristol Approach to Living with Cancer*, *The Tibetan Book of Living and Dying*, *The Ten-Minute Life Coach*, the lovely Susan Love book and the Suzannah Olivier book on nutrition, as well as about five others, some of which I have not even looked at. The self-help industry has done very well out of me and my cancer, thank you very much.

They are all good books, BUT there is a part of me that is moving on from cancer and all that it has meant in my life. I know I have not even finished my treatment yet, and that I have a mammogram next week which once was so daunting I did not think I would be able to stay sane for six weeks waiting for it, and then suddenly (partly because of 'project vantastic') I forgot about it as I was getting on with my life.

I became too busy to worry about my cancer because my static caravan needed kitting out. I suppose the doctor was right, the one who said, 'You will get on with living your life and only think about it around the time of your check-ups.' When she told me that, I thought she was slightly blasé and a little bit bonkers if she thought this wasn't going to be occupying my every waking thought for the rest of my life.

It is a little bit like a lover who cheated on you. You hate them and everything they have done to you, but the time you spent with them has shaped you and is part of you and it can't be undone. So as much as you feel let down and betrayed by them, that happening makes you stronger and, when you have finished the grieving that goes with that relationship ending, you come out the other end a stronger person determined to go on to bigger and better things.

That might be the worst analogy on the planet, but it's as if I've done my grieving. I have searched so deep into my soul that I despaired of what I found there at times, but at other times I came upon a strength and courage that I didn't know I possessed, and both of those things together are very powerful.

So although I have used my self-help books, and no doubt there may be times when I may need to return to them, to remind myself of where I was and where I am going, I shall take them away from my bedside, dust them down and put them away in a drawer for another day.

March 21, Wednesday

I am SO excited! I rang the caravan people and told them the cheque would be available to cash next Monday and could we bring some stuff down and they said yes, so I asked if we could stay the night. I said, 'I'm good for the money,' to Bob who replied, 'OK, as long as you don't come down and get drunk.' Bloody hell, hope he doesn't have a webcam in there. So I rang Julia and asked if she could come with her big estate car so we could get all the stuff down in one go, as there is no way it will all fit into our car. So she is coming with Lloyd and helping with the stuff. I can't believe it, I know it's only a caravan but it feels like out of all this I have done something that I have always wanted to do.

I have always wanted to have a place in Tenby. God, it's my dream to retire there, and now I dare to believe that I might actually do that with Rhodri, growing old, and waiting for him to go grey with me.

Here I am now, in debt and probably will be broke for a few years, but I have a place to go in Tenby with my children who sometimes do and sometimes don't drive me mad.

I have asked Martyn for five extra unpaid weeks off a year. He has agreed and I realise I would never have asked if I hadn't had cancer. I would have feared that my colleagues would think I was not committed to my work. I am committed to my work, and I work very hard, but I need to spend this time with my children. I will never get it back: once they have grown up it will be too late to sit on beaches and in seaside cafés. Too late to spend hours on end outside looking in rock pools and walking in fields, so I am going to do it now, not when I've got the money because it will be too late then.

I am going to capture this moment in time with my two growing children who make me smile and laugh and who never fail to amaze me with their wonder of the world and the thoughts they share with me as they make sense of it.

Also with my husband who has stood by me and loved me for the person I am in dark times, when I have been difficult to live with, and irrational, and ill. He has become a man, a very fine man, the man I always thought he could be. And I will be able to take the time we all spend together in our caravan and bottle it all up and put it in my head and it will be mine for ever to keep there.

Pip came round last night with her new man, Jason, who was very likeable. I said to Rhodri before they came, 'God, Rhods, all these women having new men, I feel like I'm missing out on something,' and I could tell he didn't like it, so I kissed him really passionately on the lips to show him I didn't mean it, and it was a really lovely kiss, just like we used to have in the old days when we first met, and I thought, We've still got a bit of that magic.

Took Elis to the optician's for the second time; he is complaining about colours in front of his eyes. I told her his first language wasn't Welsh so some of the letters he might pronounce differently. I was half-convinced he was doing it in order to get glasses. She put some drops in his eyes, which confirmed what he was saying about his vision in one eye, apparently. I tried to get him to read his schoolbooks when we got in, and he made out he couldn't see, which is very funny as he has managed to read them for the last two years.

Anyway it turns out he does need glasses, which I never expected: the optician says he needs them for reading and close-up work. She explained all this to me and I asked her to explain it to Elis. I don't like it when people talk about your children as if they are not in the room, or couldn't possibly understand, so she told him he had to wear glasses and I thought, God, he's going to cry, because when I was in school it was a bit of a stigma to wear glasses and children were basically ridiculed – although not by me, of course, as I was perfect. She said to him, 'Do you have any questions to ask me?' He looked thoughtfully for all of twenty seconds, going, 'Umm . . .' and then he said, 'Do you think I will need to wear them playing tag?' She thought he could manage without them for tag. Then the man who measured his eyes said, 'Are you OK with wearing glasses?' Elis said that he was and the man asked Elis to choose some frames so he went for a rather bright blue pair with Pepsi written on the side (Elton John eat your heart out, I thought). I tried to persuade him to have something a little more low-key, but he wanted the bright blue (blue for Bluebirds – aka Cardiff City) Pepsi ones as you would if you were seven and completely bombarded with Pepsi marketing.

So I agreed. After all, he has to wear them. We were in the car and I said, 'You don't mind wearing glasses, Elis, do you?' and he said, in a very grown-up voice, 'Why would I mind wearing glasses? At last, I can see.' I felt a bit guilty for doubting his eye test. The glasses will be ready next week and I have warned Rhodri, on pain of death, that if he ever, ever mentions anything derogatory about Pepsi and commercialism and puts Elis off wearing glasses, he will have me to answer to.

March 22, Thursday

Oh, thank the Lord for the credit card. How would we function without it? Our whole economy is predicated on credit so I will NOT feel guilty about using it. I have done a major Argos shop for caravan essentials – mini-Hoover, microwave, smoke alarms, clothes airers, bedding, kettle, toaster, sandwich-maker, hairdryer – although Rhodri asked me why I needed one. I explained rather huffily that I would need one again one day. So, together with my IKEA purchases I have everything one could possibly need to equip one's caravan. I don't think I have left anything out. God knows, I've spent enough time making lists and doing price comparisons. I am getting slightly nervous as we only saw the caravan for about ten minutes and now I am thinking it is a bit tatty and wasn't quite what I wanted. It's madness, I've spent weeks finding the cheapest bedding and electrical items and only ten minutes buying the bloody caravan. Buying our house was even worse; we had only been in one room and I told Rhodri to put an offer on it. We did so on the strength of the garden; we hadn't even been upstairs and the house needed so much work doing to it. I had said I would only move into a house where everything was done as Osh was only two weeks old and all I wanted to do was move my stuff in and decorate, but within less than ten minutes we'd made the biggest purchase of our lives on the strength of a lovely garden on a sunny day. It's still a lovely garden on a sunny day. It's perfect, and the house fits us. It's true about getting a feeling about a place the minute you walk in. Let's hope the same applies to caravans.

March 23, Friday

Rhodri is on a works night out tonight; Michael is leaving to go and do *Songs of Praise*, so instead of doing what I said to myself I would be doing, which is to sort my caravan stuff out and have an early night, I go to the shops to buy the children chips and myself a bottle of wine. I then have chips with them, put them to bed, open the wine and spend the night drinking most of it and ringing practically everyone I know on the planet, for a chat.

March 24, Saturday

'Project vantastic' has arrived and, like every other major event that happens in my life, I have a little bit of a hangover. Why I couldn't wait until all this stuff was loaded, unloaded and in its place is beyond me, but here I am with two cars full of stuff to sort out and all I want is to go to sleep. Ate cheese on toast and a Big Mac and Coke, so felt a little bit better when I got there.

March 25, Sunday

The caravan is perfect! Yes, just like houses, my gut feeling is right; it is not in the least bit tatty, it is all lovely and squeaky clean and tidy and enormous with loads of space for everything. It took us most of the day to unpack all the stuff and find homes for it. Rhodri took the children to the park so Julia and I set to work on a few things, then Julia took Lloyd and Elis swimming while Rhodri, Osh and I unpacked more stuff; by the evening it was more or less done.

Julia, who is a caravan veteran, took Lloyd and Elis to the club in the evening and they did games and had a bit of a disco there so they were both very happy. Osh wouldn't go to bed until about ten. I have to say though, I don't think I have been so cold in a long time. Julia tells me in the morning that they always leave the heating on at night in their van.

The last time I was in a caravan it was Mediterranean weather so I was a little unprepared, trying to find the switch for the heating at two in the morning without waking three children up, so I put two jumpers on. Osh woke at 6.30, argh, think he must have been cold. I know I was bloody freezing so I got up with him and went into the living room and put the gas fire on. I wasn't going to use the gas fire as I thought it was too dangerous around the children, but have had second thoughts now. I realise I will need it so will buy a guard for next time and be in heated luxury.

Elis went off to the little park by himself: it was a HUGE moment for me. I said to Rhodri, 'I really want to give him some freedom and this is a good place to do it, plus I get a bit of head space, but while I am trying to savour the headspace I keep thinking about one hundred things that he might be doing or that might happen to him.' Rhodri said, 'That's the dilemma of a modern parent', as if he'd been reading some book or something.

So I secretly went to check on Elis a few times, then took Osh for a walk and I kept thinking every time we did something like go to the beach, We wouldn't be doing this in Cardiff, or when I went for a long walk I was thinking to myself, I wouldn't be going for a walk in Cardiff, as if Cardiff is the Bronx or something, but for two days I had been outside more with the children than I had been in months.

Elis has a bit of freedom and has already made a new best friend, Patrick. Osh ran around until he fell asleep and I even managed to read a paper and have a bit of 'me' time. It was a fantastically sunny weekend and Rhodri kept saying, 'I can't believe we've got this caravan,' and I was glad because I think I bulldoze him into doing things, but this time we were both so happy with our lovely new caravan and all was right with the world.

March 26, Monday

Osh is at my feet while I write this. I was wondering why I have never written my diary with Osh around, and now I remember – it's because he won't let me. I said, 'You are so cute,' and he said, 'No, I'm not, I'm Oshy.'

I have been a busy bee today. I am supposed to be revising for my Welsh exam but have yet to do a thing. Instead, I got the garden furniture out of the shed, sanded it down and painted it with teak oil, washed the patio and mowed the lawn. The garden looks lovely and the sun is shining and I'd rather be pulling out my own teeth with a pair of pliers than studying. I will do it tomorrow.

Rachel, the student who is following me, came to see me today for the last time while I had my radiotherapy session. She is revising for proper exams to be a doctor – not very easy. I could probably pass the Welsh exam that I am doing on very little work. She is going to be on the wards soon, diagnosing people's illnesses. She is very young; even she thinks she is young to be doing this, but I have every faith in the medical profession after my recent encounters with it and I have every faith in her abilities.

She told me that in medical school, they say in the future that cancer will not be seen as a life-threatening disease, but a chronic disease because they would have mastered how to cure it, or at least keep it at bay. I found that quite reassuring because I hope that with all the advances in breast cancer treatment, there will be women whose lives will be saved and who, like me, can dare to think about a future after breast cancer, a future that is long and happy.

March 27, Tuesday

I went to the clinic today to see the same doctor I saw a few weeks ago, the one who freaked me out talking about secondary cancers. It is amazing what a few weeks and a bit of sunshine can do for you, because I felt completely different when I spoke to her. I was discussing the options of having my ovaries out and mentioned that someone said I could have genetic testing. She said she would not recommend me for genetic testing because there is nothing to suggest I have it with my history. We talked about my periods and ovaries, and she advised me not to have my ovaries out, but to take Tamoxifen and see what happens with regards to the menopause. She said that Tamoxifen can stop my periods, as I am worried about those heavy periods

I had while I was on chemo. I could not go out to work like that, so I would have had something done about them, but I guess I will wait and see what happens.

The most interesting thing she said was that Tamoxifen will not only stop oestrogen going to the site of my tumour, but it will also stop it going to any rogue cells that have left the tumour, and that could be in my body: it just stops them growing.

At this point I thought, Yes, thank you, I will have some of that. It sounds good to me. So next Thursday, the day after my radiotherapy, I start taking Tamoxifen. I asked her what happens now with regards to my treatment and she gave me a slip of paper to make an appointment in a year's time.

As of next Wednesday, I am out of the system for a year, unless I get any problems, of course. I'm not sure what I expected – a leaving party with balloons – but I have been in the system for so long and it is so intensive that suddenly next Wednesday that's it, no more appointments, no more treatments, just take my tablet every day for the next five years and go back once a year for a mammogram to make sure nothing sinister is lurking there. It seems strange, I've waited for this moment for so long and next Wednesday I will be cast adrift on my own in the world and I will have my life back again and I hadn't really thought about it.

I went to see Rosie; my flushes and sweats have completely stopped and I am convinced it is the acupuncture, because as soon as I started having it again they stopped.

On the way I had Red Dragon radio on in the car and was singing along and I thought, God, I haven't had a music station on for years other than Radio Three. The sun was shining and my window was down and I was singing my head off and it felt bloody great to be alive. Rosie loved my new hair and red lipstick. I have gone commando – my wig has gone into retirement!

I dyed my hair last night and went to the garage to get petrol without my wig on. Out of the context of the cancer hospital I will look like someone with very short hair, not someone who has had chemotherapy. I have been grateful for my wig and I feel almost as if I am being disloyal, leaving it behind. My hair is still very short but I have had enough of hiding behind my wig. I want my own hair back. I don't really care any more what people will think of my hair. I asked Rhodri and he said I looked fine and it wasn't too short, but it is very short so I asked the most brutally honest person in the house – Elis – and he said, 'Mum, you look fine,' and I knew if I didn't he would tell me – he has no agendas. Short as it is, I just think I have battled with cancer and I have come through the other end. The last thing in the world I am worrying about is whether people will be looking at my hair and thinking it is too short.

I am a cancer survivor. I've said it – *I have survived cancer* – and now I am crying because up until this point I have been terrified of even thinking that. I am going to live, I am NOT going to be a statistic.

March 28, Wednesday

Christine, Elis's childminder, is also having radiotherapy at the moment at the same clinic as me. I have been seeing her most mornings with Steve her husband. Before Christine came to the clinic I didn't speak to anyone else. This isn't because I am stand-offish or anything but merely because I do not like people telling me about their illnesses. Not that I don't care, of course I do, but it frightens me, in truth.

I assumed that the women were in for breast cancer but they do all types of cancers and the lady I spoke to, when we were waiting for two hours once when they had forgotten about us, told me intimate details of her cancer which was in her rectum. I then went away thinking, God, you can get cancer in your rectum. I don't know why I thought you couldn't, because you can get it anywhere presumably. Then I thought, That's one more cancer to worry about.

So, if I don't speak to people then I won't know what is wrong with them and we can all be blissfully unaware of the horrible 'other' cancers lurking out there, that we would only worry about. However, since Christine has come to the clinic we are discussing the intricate details of our cancers and putting the world to rights. Christine does her knitting and we chatter away for all the world as if we are waiting for a bus and not having radiotherapy in order to save our lives.

Elis has had his glasses. On the way to pick them up he said, 'I've changed my mind. I don't want the Pepsi ones any more, I want the plain ones.' I explained that they had made the Pepsi ones especially for him and he couldn't change his mind. I have bought a spare pair for him, which are plain, because I thought he'd break the Pepsi ones; something would happen to them, guaranteed. I didn't realise that the 'something' would be before we had even left the car park. He managed to slide off the piece that goes over your ears, leaving a potentially fatal spike, so I had to go back and get them to heat it up and put it back on. I now have to write to Miss Smith, Elis's teacher, to explain that he has to wear them.

Rhodri and Elis went to the Wales v San Marino (don't know where that is, probably should) match in the Millennium Stadium with Alison and Jay and Peter and Jonah. Wales won, so they were triumphant upon return.

March 29, Thursday

I had my mammogram today. The day I thought would be a lifetime coming came and went. It was quite painful on the breast that I am having radiotherapy on, but apart from that it was fine. I was desperately trying to look at the images but couldn't see them. I have an appointment in two weeks for the results as I am away at the caravan the week they will get them. I figure that if anything was wrong Gill would call me, but maybe it doesn't work like that. I might ring and ask her to call me with the results, otherwise I'll be worrying on my holidays and it will just be another thing hanging over me until I know the results.

March 30, Friday

Elis had a sleepover at Ben's house, so it was just me, Rhodri and Osh. We were going to get a Chinese takeaway but decided to go to the restaurant we went to on my birthday. I thought it was slightly mad after our last trip, but was prepared to give it a go. Osh was perfection. If you told him not to do something, he didn't, he sat and ate and we had a really nice time. I think Elis and Osh wind each other up in restaurants.

Apparently I am an inspiration, which is always good to know. There's another woman having radiotherapy and I was waiting in the inner room ready for my turn and she came out and didn't have her wig on. It's a bit like mine, but blonde. It took me a few seconds to register who she was without her wig. She said, 'Your hair is fantastic.' I said, 'Thanks. I was just so fed up with wearing that wig, I want my own hair back now.' She asked me if her hair was shorter than mine and I thought it was actually a bit longer. 'You've inspired me to go without it,' she said. Yeah, sisters doing it for themselves!

March 31, Saturday

I was supposed to go to a Welsh away-day today but I
didn't go. I am so tired and didn't get to bed until late, and
Osh didn't get up until about nine, which was great, so I
just couldn't get out of bed. I am feeling very tired at the
moment. It does take its toll on you, the radiotherapy, I just
want it to be all over – and it will be, next Wednesday. I
want my life free of hospital appointments and treatments. I
want to get my strength back together in preparation for
returning to work. I've got nine weeks after the
radiotherapy finishes to do this.

Before I had my treatment, I was wondering if it was too
long, but now I don't think so. It takes about two to three
weeks after the treatment finishes for the effects to wear off,
so then I'll have just over a month to get back to normal
again.

My breast is very painful now; it's not excruciating but
if you poked it I would probably be on the ceiling. It feels
rather like when your breast milk is drying up; it is very red
and has a rash on it, but all in all it's bearable, especially as
I know that in about two weeks it will start to settle down.

I don't think I'll be able to take Elis swimming though,
when I'm in Tenby on my own as I'm worried that the rash,
which has some sores on it, might get infected.

Osh has gone up to the farm; my mother is going to look
after him while I do my Welsh day, as Rhodri and Elis are
going to watch Cardiff together tomorrow. I ended up
taking Osh up there and then going on a charity shop trawl
with my mother – our favourite pastime.

April 1, Sunday

I hadn't realised it was April Fools Day or I would have
been larking about all morning. Took Elis to Llandeilo to

Owain's house. Rhodri's parents met us there to take him up to Aberystwyth for a week's holiday. Rhodri has man's flu and while I know I should try to be a bit more tolerant, I do find it very difficult. I think I've gone through months of cancer treatment and hardly ever complained (I am a martyr); he gets a cold and everybody knows about it.

He was like a bear with a sore head and said he couldn't possibly drive to Llandeilo and that there was no point him going and in any case he was too ill. So I ended up taking Elis myself, which I didn't really want to do, as it's two hours' driving and I am very tired. Eva was not there and Rhodri's mother said she was on a hen night. Owain corrected her and said it wasn't a hen night; the woman was going to get married yesterday but had found out that the boyfriend had been having an affair. So the wedding was called off and they all met up on the day to have a girls' night out. Rhodri's mother wasn't so sure it was a good idea and asked me what I would do. I said, 'I would thank my effing lucky stars I'd had such a lucky escape and be dancing in the street, especially after leaving my miserable git of a husband this morning.' I actually forgot for a moment there he was her son, but she found it amusing anyway. Elis was raring to go off with them.

Osh was coming back this afternoon; however, my mother put him in the car and as my father was about to drive off, he threw up everywhere so my mother is keeping him up there until Wednesday when my treatment finishes. Rhodri pulled a face at this.

I said, 'OK, we'll get him back and when I have my treatment you can come back and look after him.'

'Better leave him there then,' he said. Heaven forbid he should have to look after his own child.

271

April 2, Monday

Went to Richard E's house last night. One of the programmes they worked on in the summer was on the telly so they had a bit of a get-together with the people who made the programme. It was all really lovely and the food was the most fantastic I have ever tasted. Richard's wife, Monserrat, is Catalan and cooks these amazing dishes. I am salivating thinking about it. I have invited them over for lunch in the next few weeks. Not quite sure how I can compete – well, actually I just can't, so will have to think of something lovely to prepare – or something lovely for Rhodri to prepare as I will grudgingly admit that he is a better cook than me; plus if it is not nice, Rhodri has cooked it, not me.

When Rhodri woke up this morning, I was sitting at the computer reading the news on-line. 'How are you feeling today, Rhods?' he said out loud. I, having completely forgotten about his man's flu, especially as he was knocking back the drinks at Richard's and was the life and soul of the party, said, 'Oh, yes, how are you feeling today?' He went into a laborious description of how he is actually feeling which, in truth, I am not actually interested in, then said, at the end, sarcastically, 'Thanks for asking.' So I lost my patience and said, 'I've just gone through bloody chemotherapy for four months and I don't recall you asking me every day how I was.' He ignored this as he knows I will always out-trump him on illness, or will bring out childbirth which he can never ever, compete with, but I duly toddled off to the shop to get him some Lemsip because nothing else would do, apparently

Without two children in the house, Rhodri and I went for a long walk by the river in the evening; it was lovely and sunny. I had put one of his jumpers on and have to admit that, without my red lippy and with his man's top, I did look like a bloke. I have come to terms with the fact that I

272

am never going to look like the pint-sized princess of pop, so I will just have to live with me and will my hair to grow quickly.

April 3, Tuesday

Tomorrow is my last radiotherapy appointment; after nearly nine months of treatment it is finally going to be over. When you are going through it, right in the middle of it, all you feel is that it is never-ending. You are wishing the days away because each day means one less of having to walk down those long corridors, seeing all those sick people, knowing that you are one of them.

I used to think that perhaps people thought I was one of the staff, not one of the patients, not one of the people with cancer, but now my hair is so short that in a cancer hospital I couldn't be anything else. I am still quite young to be there as a lot of people are much older than me, but I am one of them and will stand alongside them because I am proud of myself to have come through this. I don't need to pretend that I am not a cancer patient because I am, and although it has been bloody hard I've come through the other end.

So I will hold my head up high and look the world in the face and smile a great big bloody smile because cancer has changed me for ever and I will NOT be afraid of it.

April 4, Wednesday

My treatment has finished. For nine months of my life I've wanted this day to come. Nine months – the same amount of time you carry a baby, but with different expectations at the end. Or maybe not so different because a baby is a new life and for me this will be *my* new life – a rebirth, if you like.

I was so happy going to the hospital today, knowing the months of being treated, the sickness, the anguish, the fear would be over on THIS DAY. And on THIS DAY I would get my life back again.

I no longer have to plan my days around hospital appointments and treatments. It felt so weird, knowing this was it. I went in and the staff were their usual chatty selves. I gave them a box of Roses and said, 'Thanks very much for zapping me.'

They are all so lovely! The staff at the hospital have a vocation and are really rather special people. They did their final zapping and we said our goodbyes and that was it, it was over.

I go back in two weeks for a check on my breast and the results of the mammogram, and then I do not have to come here for another year. Just over nine months of being treated for breast cancer and it is finished.

I left the hospital wanting to jump in the air, I was so happy, and I got in the car and put the radio on and I was beaming; I must have looked the picture of happiness if anyone could have seen me. As I drove off I started singing along to a song on the radio. I can't remember what it was – I just know I was singing at the top of my voice, smiling away, and the next thing I knew, I was crying. It was just a tear or two at first and then before I knew it I was sobbing, great enormous sobs wracking my body, and I had to pull over into a side street because I was crying so much I couldn't see.

I sat in the car slumped over the wheel and sobbed and sobbed until there was nothing left. I cried because the fucking nightmare was over and I didn't have to pretend any more.

April 15, Sunday

I have just returned from ten days at the caravan with Rhodri, the children, and Sioned and Ali for some of the time. I spent the first three days arguing with Rhodri, then my period started. So I am not yet infertile: despite everything my body has gone through, I still have periods. It never ceases to amaze me how resilient the human body is.

I realised when Rhodri had gone home, and I was on my own with the children for a week, that I tend to view any argument or negative incident between us as if there is something fundamentally dysfunctional about our relationship. I need to realise that people do have rows, they are part of everyone's relationships. I know that if I am pre-menstrual I have a very negative view of Rhodri – I will watch out for that in future. It is not him who changes, it is me.

Elis has a new lease of life. He found a friend Dylan, and for ten days they were inseparable. He has blossomed with his newfound freedom. He is able to ride around on his bike and go to the park, as long as he comes back to check with us now and again, and is not out when it is dark. He is really responsible; I realised that he has never had the opportunity to take much responsibility in his life up to now because when we are in Cardiff we are with him 24/7.

Osh was my little doting pal all holiday; like Elis and Dylan we were inseparable. I've felt a bit low since I came back this afternoon and I'm not sure why. I had such a fantastic ten days and the sun shone non-stop. I thought the children might be too much for me, but they weren't, they were so good. I just loved every minute of being on holiday with them; they are such wonderful small human beings and I've missed them over the last nine months.

God, I've missed them.

I want to hold them in my arms for ever and ever, and never let them go. I think when we were down at the caravan, for the first time in months, with just me and my babies and with the sun shining, it was as if nothing had ever touched my life.

It was as if the cancer had never happened. I think I had forgotten what life was like before I had cancer. Being down at the caravan and feeling so well, I feel I have moved on and, moving on, I fear going back again, or maybe I fear going forward.

I have been in a bubble, a cocoon, for so long that the thought of going back into the real world of work is daunting.

I became friendly with Dylan's nan Doreen and she looked so much like my own grandmother. I cried once when I thought about her. And I thought about my nanna Pitcher, who has died now, and I wanted her back there and then. My lovely calming grandmother with the reassuring touch. I wanted her to hold me in her arms and tell me she loved me, like she used to when I was a little girl. But I am not a little girl any more; at least not in years or looks, but there is a little girl still inside me who is afraid and sad sometimes, and needs someone to put their arms around her, just like I do with my babies, and tell her everything is going to be all right. I just want everything to be all right in my life.

April 16, Monday

Today is my little Oshy's birthday. My not-so-little boy is three. He doesn't really understand the concept of birthdays and kept giving me his presents and saying, 'It's your birthday, Mum.' Every time he had a gift he would say so sincerely, 'Thank you very much.' He is so cute; he had a Scooby Doo cake and candles and he blew them out twice because he loved it so much the first time. I am so, so lucky to have two wonderful, healthy, beautiful children.

April 17, Tuesday

I had my mammogram results today and everything is fine. I am so relieved it is finally over. I have told all my friends and family and people at work, and everyone is so happy for me. For once I do feel that I can be happy, and that this is news worth celebrating. I am not cured, they do not use that word, but I am in remission. I will be monitored for at least the next five years and I will be on Tamoxifen for five years and have a mammogram every year. I am not going to let cancer blight my life with worry and wonder what might happen and if it might come back.

I am going forward thinking that it will NOT come back, and I will not be frightened to say that. I am asking the Cosmos for my health, and with a bit of help from me along the way, I am hoping the Cosmos will give it right back to me.

I do not want my cancer to come back. I want to be cured and never to have to face this again. The fear is there, of course, and at times it can haunt you and I guess I could be small and quiet and hope that it will pass me by and not notice me again and let me live a peaceful life with Rhodri and my two boys.

But to do that would be doing a disservice to myself, because for all the darkness that it has brought to me, cancer has also brought me light. My cancer has changed me and shaped me into the person I have become.

Cancer has made me confront demons in my life that I would never have otherwise had the courage to confront. Cancer has shown me angels in the form of the people who have cared for me, and my family and friends who have stood by me and loved me. It has brought me together with my husband in a way I would never have thought possible. We started off two very different people in one place and now I feel that we are as one, united, and I would never have thought that would happen.

I thought that we might crumble, but we did not, we became stronger. My eyes half-closed to life are open because of cancer. I have made decisions that I would never otherwise have made.

So I will NOT lead the small quiet life I envisaged at some points along this journey, living in fear of cancer. I AM going to live a large and loud life, full of love and happiness with my three boys, Rhodri, Elis and Osian. I will shout at the top of my voice that I am alive and, no matter what is to come in the future, whatever life throws at me, I will catch it and throw it back and like Aslan the great lion in Narnia, I will come back the stronger person because of it.

It is the end of a beautiful sunny day. The sun is setting and the sky is streaked with red. I've bathed my two boys. Elis is downstairs with his father watching the cricket and despite the fact that I've asked them to keep the noise down, they can't contain themselves and keep shouting out, their voices carrying throughout the house.

Osh can hear them and even though he can hardly keep his eyes open, he wants to go and be with them. So I take him in my arms and breathe in his smell and even though he is three years and nearly one day old he lies still like a baby. While I cradle him in my arms he looks up at me and I look back at him and I rock him gently. I'm sitting on my bed watching the sun set, glad to be alive, and there is nowhere on earth at this moment in time that I would rather be.

About the author...

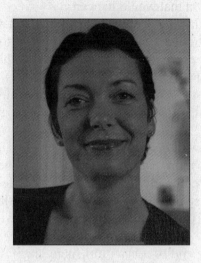

Michelle Williams-Huw was born in 1967 in Pontypool. She lives in Cardiff with her husband and two children aged three and seven. She has worked in the film and television industry in Cardiff for the last eleven years and has worked for BBC Wales for the last five years.

For more information please visit
www.michellewilliams-huw.com

For more information about Accent Press
titles please visit

www.accentpress.co.uk